Recipes & Diet Advice for Endometriosis

Updated/Improved

Carolyn Levett

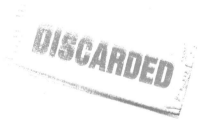

Recipes & Diet Advice for Endometriosis

Updated/Improved

By

Carolyn Levett

The publication of this book is supported by

www.endo-resolved.com

**The motivational advice website for women and girls
who suffer from the disabling disease of Endometriosis**

We can heal ourselves beautifully and the body does a brilliant job if it is given the chance. To quote from Deepak Chopra from Quantum Healing.

'..........we already know that the living body is the best pharmacy ever devised. It produces diuretics, painkillers, tranquillisers, sleeping pills, antibiotics, and indeed everything that is manufactured by the drug companies, but it makes them much, much, better. The dosage is always right and given on time; side effects are minimal or nonexistent; and the directions for using the drug are included in the drug itself, as part of its built-in intelligence.'

Every five days our whole intestinal lining is renewed. You make a new liver every 6 weeks. A new skin once a month. Every six months we have a new bloodstream. A complete new set of bones within 2 years. Even our brain cells are replaced. The DNA that holds memories of millions of years of evolution, even that is replaced every six weeks.

Now let's see if we can kick start your body to repair and renew itself!

Other books by this author:

Reclaim Your Life – Your Guide towards Healing of Endometriosis -

A motivational, practical and informative book to inspire confidence in your ability to heal form Endometriosis.

Books published and supported by:

www.endo-resolved.com

Dedication

This book is dedicated to all the women and girls in the world who suffer from the disabling disease of endometriosis. Their stories of pain, distress and suffering that were sent to the website at Endo-Resolved, led me to write this practical resource to assist them have a carefully planned diet that would help to alleviate the symptoms and pain of endometriosis.

With thanks:

I would like to thank firstly all those women who have taken the time to send me their feedback, having read the previous edition of this book, and given me tips or ideas of what they would like to see included in a book about diet for endometriosis. Thank you. And to my partner, who is a highly qualified and experienced chemist, who has given me advice on all the complex topics relating to chemistry and chemicals.

Disclaimer: The material in this book is intended as an educational tool to offer information about your options available for a diet for Endometriosis. The advice in this book is intended solely for informational and educational purposes only and not as medical advice. Please consult a medical professional if you have questions about your health.

Forward

When I had endometriosis, (and I emphasize <u>had</u>, to encourage you that you can repair the body before we go any further) I used my intuition. I used it with the aim to help me eradicate the disabling disease of endometriosis and choose my own course of action to repair my body.

I didn't 'catch it' from someone else, I wasn't born with it, so I knew deep down it was totally possible for my body to heal.

After the initial shock of being diagnosed with the worst case of endometriosis my gynaecologist had ever seen, and being given my treatment options based on drug therapy, it was then that I decided to follow my own path for healing with safe treatments. I did lots of research and I talked to friends and other sufferers. Fortunately many of my friends were very in-tune or knowledgeable about using natural treatments, and thankfully I had plenty of advice and support from these friends.

After seeking advice, I decided the best course of action was to improve the focus of my diet, which already being mainly vegetarian, simply required that I omitted certain foods that I knew were not suited for optimum nutrition and exclude any food weaknesses I had like sugar and dairy. Additionally I chose to use homeopathy with the support of a talented homeopath to assist my healing. I also included various natural treatments and beneficial measures like meditation, essential oils, and dietary supplements; and I even went to see a couple of healers (sometimes just to give me spiritual and emotional support).

It did take a long time – *but I healed and I was given proof of this by my gynaecologist*. It was a struggle sometimes, and yes, I did have times of despair like many other women who suffer this disease – BUT I NEVER GAVE UP.

It is not my aim here to provide my own endometriosis story as that has already been written elsewhere in my accompanying book 'Reclaim Your Life – Your Guide to Aid Healing of Endometriosis'.

This book has been put together to help other sufferers by providing a comprehensive diet and nutrition resource that they can utilize to help with their own symptoms and support them on their own journey towards healing the body.

Based on personal experience of recovery from endometriosis, backed up with training in Nutritional Therapy and Aromatherapy (studies I undertook when I regained my health); combined with positive feedback from past readers and messages sent to the website, this *new edition* has been put together to improve and build on that advice – written with passion and thorough research.

With healing thoughts

Carolyn Levett - BA Hons, Dip NT

Contents

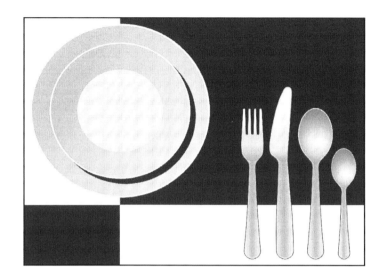

Introduction

**Welcome to your diet and recipe resource
to help you combat Endometriosis**

The focus of this diet …..

The diet for endometriosis is focussed on reducing your symptoms, boosting your immune system and helping you to obtain healing from this disease.

Many people are beginning to realise the link between health and the food they eat. This can apply to physical as well as emotional health. Research is beginning to discover that emotions and behaviour can also relate to food intake and this has been highlighted by hyperactivity in children. And unfortunately, obesity has become the modern epidemic of the Western world due to really dreadful diets.

Fortunately, the belief that diet can improve health and reduce the risk of a number of serious diseases has become a proven fact by clinical research. It's a pity that many of our doctors do not have the same opinion or interest - but that's medical training for you.

Short term and long term diets can be designed to help with certain health issues like diabetes, candida, and food intolerances. You can also achieve great health benefits with a special diet for Endometriosis.

As well as improving your immune system, you will also be able to balance your hormones, get rid of unwanted oestrogen, increase your energy and obtain additional health benefits.

Diet is a great way to start taking control for your own health. It's also a great way for you to monitor what is happening to your body and to monitor your symptoms. Just making changes to certain foods, or by omitting certain food groups, you can learn what is causing your symptoms.

The proof is in the pudding …….

There are many women who are seeing vast improvements in their symptoms of the disease by using diet and good nutrition. Some women are seeing results within a matter of 2 to 3 weeks, with a huge reduction of the symptoms of pain, a reduction of inflammation, reduction of pain with their periods, less intestinal problems and an increase in energy levels. *(Read some of the testimonials further on.)*

Some of the health improvements reported by sufferers who have followed the diet include:

- Reduction in endometriosis pain
- Reduction of inflammation in the abdominal cavity
- Reduction of intestinal problems and Irritable Bowel symptoms
- Reduction of problems relating to Candida
- Reduction of bloating and better digestion
- Reduction of pain during menstruation
- Improved fertility and pregnancy success
- Improved energy levels
- Improvement with constipation
- Improved eye sight / improved skin
- Weight loss – which will reduce stored oestrogen in the fatty tissues

These are just the main improvements and I am sure there will be others.

You will no doubt have read over and over again (via the internet and in other books) of all the food groups you should leave out of your diet - and that list seems to cover many of the basic and common foods and ingredients in everyday cooking.

So this has been the driving force in putting a book like this together – to give you much needed information and guidance for this diet. **It's all very well being told what to leave OUT of your diet – but what do you put IN.**

There are loads of great recipes you can use. I have covered nearly every aspect of your diet needs here - including main meals, soups, drinks, alternatives to milk, alternatives to sugar, and alternatives to wheat for baking and cakes, puddings, sauces, dips, spreads – plus cooking tips, shopping list ideas, just to mention a few.

Additional gut health issues

And a quick note before we go onto the diet information – these recipes are about healing – to help repair many aspects of a broken body and digestive system. Therefore the recipes that have been compiled should hopefully help deal with other digestive problems which so many endometriosis sufferers seem to be dealing with, which may include:

- **Gluten/wheat/coeliac (celiac) intolerance or allergy** – gluten intolerance is divided into three distinct categories: Celiac Disease, Non-Celiac Gluten Sensitivity and a Wheat Allergy. (Technically, a wheat allergy is not intolerance to gluten).
- **Coeliac disease** – occurs when the proteins in gluten trigger your immune system to overreact with strong and unusual antibodies. Over time, the reaction caused by these antibodies wears down the villi that line the walls of your intestine (this process is called villous atrophy). These finger-like tiny hairs grab and absorb nutrients as foods pass through your lower digestive tract. As celiac disease symptoms slowly destroy these villi, you become less and less able to process any nutrition from your food. Gluten which is found in wheat, barley and rye triggers an immune reaction in people with coeliac disease. This means that eating gluten damages the lining of the small intestine. Other parts of the body may be affected – which can be diagnosed with a blood test. Some symptoms may be mistaken as Irritable bowel syndrome (IBS) or wheat intolerance.
- **Non-Celiac Gluten Sensitivity** is currently a little more difficult to pinpoint. Basically, individuals who suffer from NCGS suffer very similarly to people with Celiac Disease, but the blood test which identifies and diagnoses celiac disease returns as negative. The only way to confidently diagnose NCGS is through a gluten free diet
- **Wheat allergy symptoms** are the third category. The triggers of wheat allergy symptoms are fundamentally different from the triggers of celiac disease symptoms, but some might inaccurately refer to these symptoms as gluten allergy symptoms. This is a histamine response to wheat, much like a peanut allergy or hay fever.
- **Lactose intolerance** – milk/dairy foods – can be an issue for coeliac sufferers – can be difficult to diagnose simply based on symptoms. Hydrogen Breath Test is one method of diagnosis. The person drinks a lactose-loaded beverage and then the breath is analysed at regular intervals to measure the amount of hydrogen.
- **Irritable Bowel** – great feedback of success from past readers – unfortunately the medical profession does not actually know what causes this problem, but stress has been highlighted as the main trigger
- **Candida** – yeast overgrowth of the intestines - the candida diet is almost identical to the basis of the endometriosis diet – again the real cause/trigger is unknown – more on this later. Can be diagnosed by blood testing or stool testing.

This book is not aimed to be specifically addressing the above health / digestive issues, but it is a very good starting point, based on the problematic foods for each of these health problems. Eliminating certain food groups and keeping a diary will help you to monitor your reaction to certain foods, and to discover if you are dealing with more than one health issue.

Other possible reasons for a damaged gut!

I am not trying to alarm you here, but simply aiming to explain or highlight why your digestion may be totally 'out of whack', without going into too much detail – because essentially I want to provide solutions – not focus on problems – you get enough of those as an endometriosis sufferer. But over the course of time your gut health could have been affected by any of the following:

Bowel prep – usually taken before surgery like laparoscopy, colonoscopy. The powder that is prescribed gives the entire gut a thorough clean out – but it is so harsh it is like 'paint-stripper' for the gut. This will kill all the good bacteria in your gut and probably cause additional gut damage. (I have personal and nasty memories of this one)

Drugs – on-gong long term use of painkillers can damage the gut. Narcotic pain relievers reduce the motility of stomach contents through the digestive tract. As foods move slower through the digestive tract, excess water is removed from the contents of the colon, which makes stools dryer, sometimes resulting in constipation.

Laxatives – trying to combat constipation with laxatives can damage your intestinal flora and cause damage to the lining of your intestines. They can also make the matter worse when laxative dependency develops.

Hormone drugs – can cause many side effects relating to gut health - abdominal swelling, nausea, gastro-intestinal upsets, and liver malfunction.

Stress – this is one key issue that can really upset the natural balance of digestive enzymes, it can suppress the digestive processes, can cause inflammation, decreases natural digestive secretions, and affects contractions of your digestive muscles. Stress can also cause your colon to react in a way that gives you diarrhoea or constipation.

Therefore you can see by the list above, you need to try and address these issues, reduce these additional symptoms and try to get the gut back into balance. Reduce your use and dependency on painkillers, laxatives, hormone drugs, and try to reduce stress.

The pain, symptoms and stress of endometriosis simply becomes a downward spiral – and you will need to get on top of this, one layer at a time. Carry on reading and we can take this one step at a time.

Your digestion

The digestive system is very complex – from the moment food enters your mouth and the actions of saliva – right through to the large intestine and the final process of excretion.   There are dozens of processes, dozens of digestive enzymes, and many digestive enzymes that are still being discovered by research today.

And on top that, 80% of you immune system stems from your digestive system – so having a healthy gut is utterly vital for well-being. As I mentioned earlier, this book is not aimed at providing in-depth information about digestive health – it's about providing a practical, usable diet book, and to give you tools to help you feed yourself and heal at the same time. You will find plenty of other books to compliment this one, which will give you details about other digestive disorders.

Testimonial from Clare ....

'I bought your recipe book and went on the suggested diet about 6 months ago. In that time, I have lost 15 pounds and I feel fantastic. No more excessive gas and bloating, and my pain is virtually non-existent. I am also, finally, medication-free thanks to a terrific doctor at the New York Endometriosis and Infertility Centre. It seems that the combination of his surgical skills and your diet has been (knock-on-wood) keeping my stage 4 endo at bay. So, I want to thank you for helping me take control of my life again.'
Clare Gardner

Your Immune System – the key to your healing

This next section regarding the immune system is included in my book 'Reclaim your Life – Your Guide to Aid healing of Endometriosis'. I went into quite some detail about the immune system in that book, because this is the KEY to repairing your body. I was blown away by this discovery (below) and felt it was very valid to include it here.

There is an awful lot more to the immune system than most people realise. It now appears that the immune system goes far beyond providing protection for the body from invading organisms simply through chemical processes in the body.

I want to quote a sizeable section from a lecture given by Deepak Chopra, M.D. which is titled 'What is the True Nature of Reality? 'The Basics of Quantum Healing'. Deepak Chopra has a 'foot in both camps' regards medicine. He was born and lived in India for the first part of his life and therefore has a good understanding of Ayurvedic medicine. He later moved to the US where he has spent his career in medicine and writing.

'About 20 years ago it was discovered that our thoughts and our feelings have physical substrate to them. When you think a thought you make a molecule. To think is to practise brain chemistry. And in fact these thoughts are translated into very precise molecules known as neuropeptides. 'Neuropeptides' because they were first found in the brain; and 'peptides' because they are protein-like molecules. And thoughts, feelings, emotions and desires translate into the flux of neuropeptides in the brain.

You can think of these neuropeptides like little keys that fit into very precise locks called receptors on the cell walls or other neurons. So the way this part of the brain speaks to another part of the brain is in the precise language of these neuropeptides.

What was found subsequently, which was absolutely fascinating was that there were receptors to neuropeptides not only in brain cells but other parts of the body as well. So when scientists started looking for receptors to neuropeptides in cells of the immune system, for example: T cells, B cells, monocytes, and macrophages - when they started looking at them, they found that on the cell walls of all these there were receptors for the same neuropeptides which are the molecule substrate of thought.

So your immune cells are in fact constantly eaves-dropping on your internal dialogue. Nothing that you say to yourself, which you are doing all the time, even in sleep, escapes the attention of the immune cells. (Is that spooky or what – my words. You know what they say – careful of what you ask for because you may just get it). Not only that, the immune cells, it was subsequently discovered, make the same peptides that the brain makes when it thinks. Now here we come to a startling finding because if the immune cell is making the same chemicals that the brain is making when it thinks, then the immune cell is a thinking cell. It is a conscious little being.

In fact, the more you look at it, the more you find that it behaves just like a neuron. It makes the same chemical cords that the brain uses for emotion, thought, felling and desire. An immune cell has emotions. It has desires. It has intellect. It knows how to discriminate and remember. It has to decide when it sees a carcinogen, 'Is this a carcinogen? Should I go after it? Should I leave it alone? Is this a friendly bacteria? Should I go after it or leave it alone?' It has to remember the last time it encountered something. In fact it remembers the last time somebody else encountered the same thing.

Your immune cells can immediately recognise anything that has ever been encountered by any living species. If you are exposed to pneumococus for the first time in your life, your immune cells still remember the last time somebody somewhere in prehistoric time encountered a pneumococus and knows how to make the precise antibody to it. It is not only a thinking cell but it remembers way back into evolutionary history of not only the human species but other species as well. So you ask a good neurologist the difference between an immune cell and a neuron and they will say there isn't any. The immune cell is a circulatory nervous system.

Now if that wasn't enough of a startling discovery, the subsequent discoveries in science have been even more interesting, because when scientists started looking elsewhere in the body they found the same phenomenon. When they looked at stomach cells and intestinal cells they found the same peptides. The stomach cells make the same chemical cords that the brain makes when it thinks. Of course they are not verbally as elite as the brain, in that they don't think in English or Swahili, but nonetheless, they are thinking cells. When you say, 'I have a gut feeling about such and such,' you are not speaking metaphorically anymore. You are speaking quite literally because you're gut makes the same chemicals as the brain makes when it thinks. In fact your gut feelings may be a little bit more accurate because gut cells haven't yet evolved to the stage of self-doubt.

What science is discovering is that we have a thinking body. Every cell in our body thinks. Every cell in our body is actually a mind. Every cell has its own desires and it communicates with every other cell. The new work is not mind and body connection, we have a body-mind simultaneously everywhere.'

Do read Deepak Chopra – he is a great writer with an excellent grasp of how the body/mind works, and his books are always written with a fresh inspiring approach. I read most of his books when I was working to fix my own body. I included his quote because he talks about the intelligence of the immune system - which is also found in the digestive system – and that is what we are focussing on here.

To give you a summary of the complexities of your immune system - the major components of your immune system are:

- Thymus
- Spleen
- Lymph system
- Bone marrow
- Antibodies
- Hormones
- Digestive system
- White blood cells

I won't say any more on the immune system here. I have written an article which is available at the website about it, which describes in more detail how the immune system works and how you can support it. You will find that article here: http://www.endo-resolved.com/immunesystem.html

How to view the advice here ....

The information in this book is the bottom line, based only on ingredients and recipes that are targeted for a diet for Endometriosis and various digestive health issues in common, or relating to endometriosis. This does not mean that your diet has to be restricted to what is included here. I have not included any fish or chicken recipes - both of which can be included in your diet as long as they are from safe sources – your chicken is organic and your fish is from unpolluted waters. You don't need me to tell you how to cook your favourite protein recipes!!!

The recipes and nutritional information gives you scope to test your digestive system by eliminating certain food groups as we mentioned earlier (gluten, lactose etc). Also, you can alter and adapt many of these recipes to suit your taste. For example, if you like the sound of a particular casserole recipe but do not like xy or z vegetable, then change it to suit you. Eating food that you enjoy will also help your well-being.

This book is your bench-mark, we could not hone down your diet much lower than this otherwise you would be on a full blown detox diet. AND I want you to enjoy your food – there is even a recipe for endo-friendly chocolate here – and it has health benefits too! So enjoy your food – you will stick to the diet better and this will make you 'feel' better with the 'feel-good' factor.

Testimonial from past reader:

Mercy from USA

'Hello, I just wanted to thank you so, so much for this website. You have no idea what difference it has made in my life. I had unbearable pain from endometriosis, had laparoscopic surgery and after one year, the pains returned with a vengeance. I have been trying to get pregnant for 2 ½ yrs with no success yet I am in my twenties. I was feeling so hopeless until the day I stumbled on to this website 3 months ago.

I immediately decided to get on the Endo-diet and my first cycle after being on the diet for a month, was pain-free. I did not even need pain medication, and so was the next month, and this month as well. The other thing is since I got endometriosis my cycle has been longer than usual and for the first time in a long time I am now back on a 28 day cycle. This is the best thing that ever happened to me. Thank you for all the work you have put on this website. You have transformed my life. God bless you! And to those in endo-pain I would want to say DO NOT EVER GIVE UP! There is HOPE! Thank you.'

Hopefully you will find that these recipes do not require lots of different ingredients, or lots of complex cooking techniques. Many of the ingredients will become the basics that you should have in your food cupboard anyway. There is a shopping list near the back of the book, of items to have in your stock cupboard.

And I do know and understand how difficult it can be to undertake many daily tasks because of the symptoms of Endometriosis – I learnt that from personal experience. Many of these recipes can be cooked in bulk, and you can freeze individual portions for another day. This not only saves on your energy and effort, it also saves on your fuel bills as well.

This book is based on recipes which are:

*   wheat-free – with most being gluten free
*   lactose free
*   meat-free
*   dairy free
*   sugar-free
*   soy-free
*   additive-free
*   **but not taste free**

When are we going to start cooking I hear you say ….. well there are a few more details I want to make clear and go over before we go on to the recipes, so let's do that quickly now…………….

What has been cut out of the diet and why!

Wheat – it appears many women with Endometriosis are wheat intolerant or totally gluten intolerant. And there are some sufferers who also have Candida which is also affected by wheat/gluten. Coeliac disease and Irritable Bowel Syndrome are also on the increase especially among women with endometriosis, and the cause of these digestive problems is not really known by doctors.

It is speculated that a compromised immune system could be the trigger to any or all of the above digestive issues. It seems certain that the immune system of women with endometriosis will be under immense stress trying to combat the inflammation and implants of the disease.

When wheat has been eliminated from women's diets, in 80% of sufferers, the pain of Endometriosis has subsided and when all gluten is eliminated nearly all pain is stopped.

To Quote Dian Mills, the author of 'Endometriosis - Healing through Diet and Nutrition', 'I think there may be hormones in the wheat, or the phytic acid is locking up some of the minerals, but certainly there seems to be some modality with wheat and endometriosis. It's almost as though something within wheat that is exacerbating the implant'

The wheat that is produced today is far removed from the original crop that used to be grown many years ago. It has been altered to produce high yield crops and it is sprayed many times during the growth period. We have all seen the huge, sterile, blank expanses of modern crop fields grown today which bear no resemblance to the way crops were grown before mass, intensive farming was developed. Therefore, as a food substance it is difficult for the human digestive system to assimilate this altered crop, as well as cope with the toxic contamination caused by spraying.

Unfortunately, there are so many food stuffs that contain wheat today, especially in the West. As well as the obvious sources like breads and pastries, wheat is found in MANY convenience foods. Wheat flour is used as a thickener for many convenience dishes, in sauces and gravies, even in pharmaceuticals.

Consequently wheat and gluten can affect – endometriosis, candida, gluten intolerance, Irritable Bowel and Coeliac disease and you can now steer clear of the foods and ingredients that can cause problems, based on the recipes here.

Flour & Gluten in this book - The baking recipes in this book are nearly all gluten free, with a few recipes containing very low levels of gluten based on the type of flour/grains being used. Each recipe is marked as to whether it is gluten free or has small amounts of gluten, so you can choose which recipes to use to be safe for your personal needs.

There are many other alternatives to wheat flour for cooking and baking. A full list of different flours is covered later in the book, giving details which are gluten free, and which are related to wheat. But none of the negative flours are used in the actual recipes here.

Fortunately, there are now various companies who produce wheat-free bread, cake, muffin and pizza bases. You can buy them from your local health store or from the internet. For your own needs and taste there are recipes included here for making bread, cakes, muffins, pastry and pizzas by using alternative and safe ingredients.

Compiling recipes for the baking section has been the most difficult, to ensure they have no wheat flour/gluten, eggs, dairy, or sugar – but many of us love pizza's, pastries and pies, and that has been achieved by the selection further on.

Meat - red meat is excluded from the diet for a variety of reasons, the main reason being that red meat will increase the production of the bad prostaglandins in the body that are responsible for the production of pain messengers in the body.

- the fats in meat can contain the highest levels of dioxin in foods (dioxins convert into xeno-estrogens – chemical based oestrogens - in the body and are stored in body fat)
- animal meat increases the intake of fatty acids that stimulate the production of the prostaglandin F 2a (series 2 prostaglandins) in the body. These are partly responsible for muscle cramping, uterine cramping, pain signals and inflammation
- animal proteins produce an acid which is an inflammatory agent
- unless you eat organic meat it will be full of hormones, antibiotics and unwanted chemicals picked up through the food chain

Dairy - many vegetarians say that milk is for calves, and of course they are right. The only milk we should be ingesting is human milk as babies. But we have become so used to having milk in our diets, in many cultures around the world, but more so in the West. The use of dairy products, including milk, cheese, and butter are similar to the problems associated with meat.

- dairy products are pro-inflammatory - again caused by series 2 prostaglandins
- dairy products are not easy to digest and can interrupt the take up of other nutrients
- can be the cause of food intolerance's which can show up as illnesses like asthma, eczema and arthritis
- can cause lactose intolerance
- dairy produce is a trigger for constipation

Yoghurt - There are many sources of advice about diet for Endometriosis which advises that you do not include yoghurt in your diet. There are different types of yoghurt. It is the commercial, sweetened, flavoured yoghurts, which do need to be excluded. They are not produced using the traditional methods, they include a lot of sugar, and plenty of additives. The thinking behind this advice is that yoghurt is a dairy product, and dairy products need to be excluded from your diet, for the reasons mentioned above.

However, natural 'live' yoghurts are actually beneficial to your health. These yoghurts contain active bacteria which are beneficial to the health of your intestinal flora. These same beneficial bacteria can help you address the negative bacteria overgrowth caused by Candida.

You can buy 'live' yoghurt of various types including cow's milk yoghurt, sheep's milk yoghurt, and goat's milk yoghurt. The human digestive system does not digest milk very well, especially cow's milk. The milk that is easiest for us to digest is goat's milk, so I would advise trying goat's milk based yoghurts. It does have a distinctive strong taste, but you soon get used to it.

I have included two recipes which allow you to make alternative 'yoghurts' using nuts, so you can choose for yourself which to use. This is an area where you can test your own reaction to the different yoghurts.

Sugar - sugar is a highly refined product with concentrated carbohydrates which have a negative effect on the symptoms of endometriosis. Sugar, in all forms (refined, artificial or natural) produces a more acidic environment within the body that can encourage the inflammatory pain of endometriosis.

- sugar is another food that feeds Candida – more on candida later
- research shows that foods with a high sugar content will increase menstrual cramping as well as aggravate PMT
- it is the number one enemy of bowel movements
- causes hormone imbalances

Sugar, especially in a processed form is an immune system suppressor. Research has shown that eating 100g of sugar per day causes immune system response to be reduced by 50-60%. Sugary foods also rob the body of energy, vitamins and minerals each time they are eaten. Too much sugar in the blood stream causes the pancreas to produce insulin for its removal. This not only uses energy from the body to perform this task, but it also robs the body of vitamins and minerals, which are used to produce insulin.

Sugar encourages the overgrowth of bad intestinal flora such as candida and is therefore best avoided in any processed form. Sugar in the form of fruit should be limited to two/three pieces a day, and women with severe candida may need to reduce this still further.

Fructose / fructose mal-absorption - Fructose has not actually been omitted from the diet, but I felt it wise to include a quick mention of it here, as it can be another digestive issue that can occur – but nowhere near as frequently as gluten/coeliac/IBS issues.

Fructose is the sugar found in plants and it naturally occurs in honey, tree and vine fruits, berries and most root vegetables – for example, sweet potato. It has also been developed from sugar cane, sugar beets and corn (as high fructose corn syrup) into a cheap commercial sweetener and additive to soft drinks and processed foods.

Fructose is a rapidly fermentable sugar and it is absorbed into the wall of the small intestine, where it is used for nutrition and energy. In the case of mal-absorption, the fructose cannot be absorbed in this way and requires glucose to be present in equal amounts in order to be absorbed. If glucose is not present, the fructose will travel down to the large intestine where bacteria will cause it to ferment, releasing the gases that cause symptoms similar to those of irritable bowel syndrome (IBS) – bloating, excess wind, abdominal distension or pain, diarrhoea or constipation.

The test for fructose mal-absorption is simple – a hydrogen breath test is used to detect the gases that indicate there is unabsorbed fructose in the large intestine.

Coffee, Tea and caffeine - caffeine is found in coffee, tea and fizzy drinks and increases levels of oestrogen in the body. Coffee seems to be the biggest culprit, as it is a powerful phytoestrogen product. Drinking more than two cups of coffee daily may boost your oestrogen levels and could worsen the symptoms of endometriosis, as well as problems with breast pain.

According to researchers, women who drank the most coffee had higher levels of estradiol, a naturally occurring form of oestrogen, during the early follicular phase, or days 1 to 5 of the menstrual cycle. This increased level can be as high as 70%.

Caffeine in coffee is linked to heart disease, and coffee drinkers suffer from 60% more heart attacks than people who do not drink it. Coffee also causes palpitations, raises blood pressure and cholesterol levels, increases stomach acid secretions, aggravate fibrocystic breast disease and increases the risk of miscarriages and birth defects.

Its psychological effects include insomnia, anxiety, panic attacks and depression. Decaffeinated coffee is no better. Trichloroethylene was used to decaffeinate coffee until quite recently when it was proved to be carcinogenic. Now petrol-based solvents are often used instead, which is just as worrying. The alternatives are grain coffee made from cereals and fruits and are readily available in health-food shops.

Eggs – There are no recipes here containing eggs and egg replacers are used in their place for baking recipes. There are various reasons I have omitted them. Eggs contain oestrogen and for those of you who wish to balance your oestrogen or feel you may be oestrogen dominant then leaving out eggs will help. Also, eggs act as a binder in many cooking and baking processes, so eating too many eggs could 'bind you up' inside and cause constipation if you eat them too often.

Egg replacers can be used to bind ingredients together but they will not help the mixture to rise. If using in cakes instead of eggs it is advisable to add a little extra baking powder. Egg replacers are also readily available in health food stores.

But for those of you who wish to continue eating eggs, the levels of oestrogen obtained from one egg when used in a typical baking recipe, will be fine. But you must ensure you use only organically reared, free-range eggs. Commercially reared hens will consume hormones and chemicals in their feed which will be passed on to you.

Alcohol - Optimum liver function is essential for clearing out excess oestrogen which in turn helps to control endometriosis, as well as help your immune system fire on all cylinders. Over-consumption of alcohol is best known for causing liver damage where the liver swells with acute intoxication, sometimes painfully, and will show fatty infiltration and enlargement. Alcohol ingestion also interferes with vitamin B12 absorption. The process of eliminating alcohol from the body stresses the liver and this hinders it from expelling other toxic such as excessive oestrogen.

Yeast – Yeast is a food that causes intolerance in many people and candida is implicated as relating to yeast intolerance. Yeast related foods include yeast extract, vinegar, citric acid, stock cubes, alcohol, cheese, mushrooms, dried fruit, soy sauce.

Detoxing – physical and emotional

Undertaking a detox is the most efficient way to start any healing and repairing for the body. But I feel this is even more relevant for women with endometriosis who have used various hormone drugs and lots of pain medications. These can put untold strain on the liver, and the liver is your *key* filter for the body. Stress also causes toxins to build up in the body as stress produces many different hormones that can circulate and cause damage to the body.

Emotional detox - Personally I feel that an *emotional detox* can help immensely. We have all heard about the toxicity of our food, the air we breathe and the water we drink etc., but we don't often hear about emotional toxicity. Yet the cells of our body are actively encoded with every emotional and mental issue that has not been resolved in our lives. Different organs hold onto different emotions – so the liver is affected by anger, we can hold stress in jaw muscles which can cause severe headaches, and our stomach can churn over with stress and anxiety.

Counselling can help with detoxing our emotions. You do not necessarily need to see a counsellor for this role – any good natural therapist, whether it be a naturopath or homeopath or herbalist, can provide a good level of counselling during any treatment sessions – this role is a natural 'by-product' of the whole care and therapy process. They can then back-up this support with supplements, herbs or remedies to support the emotional side of treatment. Other helpful mechanisms to help with emotional aspects of ill health and detoxing can include massage (touch can bring up some really deep-seated emotions), and any of the other touch therapies that help to address issues of imbalances in the body. Going to see a healer will also help – ideally one that has been recommended by friends/contacts, as there are some very good healers out there.

And finally, crying has huge benefits. When you cry, the tears you produce actually get rid of specific toxins from the body as well as provide a release of the emotional 'pressure valve'. So don't be afraid to cry, or feel you are crying too often – it's good for you. I did lots of it when I had endometriosis, and one or two of the homeopathic remedies I was prescribed made me cry and shake from sobbing so deeply. Emotions seemed to be coming from the very deepest parts of my soul, and afterwards I would feel that some deeply ingrained emotions from early years, and anger about my illness were being released. So talking, touching and crying are all things you need to help you with healing.

Dietary detox – Using a very simple diet is the best way to detox, get those toxins removed from the body and give your system 'room and space' to work properly and allow the immune system to work where it is needed.

Eating a wholesome vegetarian diet encourages toxicity to be removed from the body. Certain foods like fruit will actually pull toxicity out of the cells, but not out of the body as this is done by your liver. Pulling too much toxicity out of the cells, but not out of the body is one reason people feel so ill when starting a healthy eating regime. The same effect can occur when introducing minerals in supplement form, as these also encourage toxicity to move out of cells.

It is advised when changing your diet to do so gradually and that supplements are introduced gradually. This will help you to feel more balanced and sustain you while still removing toxins from the system. There is no benefit to try and speed things up, as the liver determines how fast we detoxify.

Some individuals do a full 'fast-track' detox by going on a food fast and only eating juices for a number of days. But this can only be done if you are willing to rest for the entire time, and preferably with medical supervision, with some light exercise for maybe half an hour a day. Undertaking a full-blown detox can leave your body 'swimming' in the toxins that are being off-loaded. It is better to detox gradually through diet and eating simple foods that are going to be easy for the body to digest like fruit, steamed veg, white fish. Then you can progress onto more complex foods after a week or so of a detox plan (see further on).

The Liver and importance of looking after this vital organ

As mentioned above, your liver is a VITAL cleansing organ for the entire body. It cleans and filters everything that travels through your bloodstream. This includes toxins from food, skincare products, waste chemicals and by-products from drugs, toxins from the air you breathe, chemicals off-loaded by natural bodily processes - like releasing stress hormones that the body no longer needs after the stress has passed.

The liver also plays a vital role in flushing excess hormones from your system, as well as regulate your immune system by destroying old red and white blood cells. So your liver has a lot of work to do.

When your liver is working efficiently and coping with the amount of cleansing work required, then your body will stay in balance and you will not suffer the effects of toxic overload. This is vital for women with endometriosis, so that you can release surplus hormones and toxins, which will give the immune system the opportunity to work where it is needed – helping to tackle endometriosis.

Therefore doing a gentle and steady detox with diet will help your body and your liver to gradually off-load these toxins and allow your system to work efficiently. However, you can jump-start the detox to help cleanse your liver, which will in turn will open the 'gates' for the rest of your detox to be more effective.

How to jump-start your liver detox
Without over-loading your system

- Drink plenty of water throughout the day to 'wash out' your system
- No sugar, alcohol, caffeine, gluten – well these are all omitted from the endometriosis diet anyway so you are off to a good start
- Start the first 2 days with very clean and simple meals like salads, vegetable soups or stir fry veg – this period allows your body to adjust in readiness for the next couple of days
- After 2 days simplify the diet further for another 2 days to 'deepen' the detox – juices, raw foods like salads, steamed veg, baked veg, and herb teas
- Then for days 5 to 14 introduce whole-grains and simple protein like organic chicken and fish (if you are eating white meat).
- Get plenty of rest, some fresh air, and gentle exercise like walking during this period
- Do not use chemical based toiletries as these chemicals will be absorbed through your skin and will undermine the detox process. You need to stop using the chemical based toiletries and house-hold products anyway, to help with the long-term healing of endometriosis. You can read more about this at http://www.endo-resolved.com/toiletries.html
- You may feel sluggish and tired to start with as the toxins are off-loaded, but as the days go on you will feel more energy and more vitalised. If you continue with the simple diet regime for a

month before adding other foods to your diet, you should start to feel much more energised, and your immune system, along with the support of a healthy liver, your body will be able to really focus on dealing with your endometriosis.

Foods that will support your liver

Garlic

Just a small amount of this pungent white bulb has the ability to activate liver enzymes that helps your body flush out toxins. Garlic also holds high amounts of allicin and selenium, two natural compounds that aid in liver cleansing.

Grapefruit

High in vitamin C and antioxidants, grapefruit increases the natural cleansing processes of the liver. A small glass of freshly-squeezed grapefruit juice will help boost production of liver detoxification enzymes that help flush out carcinogens and other toxins

Beets and carrots

Both extremely high in plant-flavonoids and beta-carotene, eating both beets and carrots can help stimulate and improve overall liver function.

Green tea

This liver-loving beverage is chock-full of plant antioxidants known as catechins, a constituent known to assist the livers' overall functions. Green tea is not only delicious, it's also a great way to improve your overall diet. There is more about the benefits of green tea further in the introduction.

Leafy green vegetables

One of our most powerful allies in cleansing the liver, leafy greens can be eaten raw, cooked or juiced. Extremely high in plant chlorophylls, greens literally suck up environmental toxins from the blood stream. With their distinct ability to neutralize heavy metals, chemicals and pesticides, these cleansing foods offer a powerful protective mechanism for the liver.

Apples

High in pectin, apples hold the chemical constituents needed for the body to cleanse and release toxins from the digestive tract. This, in turn, makes it easier for the liver to handle the toxic load during the cleansing process.

Oils

Cold-pressed organic oils such as olive, hemp and flax-seed are great for the liver, when used in moderation. They help the body by providing a lipid base that can suck up harmful toxins in the body. In this way, it takes some of the burden off the liver in terms of the toxic overload that many of us suffer from.

Lemons and limes

These citrus fruits contain very high amounts of the vitamin C, which aids the body in synthesising toxic material into substance that can be absorbed by water. Drinking freshly-squeezed lemon or lime juice in the morning helps stimulate the liver.

Whole grains

Grains, such as brown rice, are rich in B-complex vitamins, nutrients known to improve overall fat metabolism, liver function and liver decongestion

Diet & Blood sugar balance

Keeping your blood sugar balance is important to assist with healing and good health. Blood sugar is all about energy and with insufficient energy the body cannot detoxify and heal. Energy is not only needed for everyday tasks, but also for the internal organs that have a job to do in keeping our bodies running smoothly. Blood sugar is also needed for the brain, otherwise you start to feel muzzy headed, develop poor concentration and suffer from depression.

Raising blood sugar levels through diet involves eating sufficient of the right kind of foods at regular intervals. It is recommended to eat six times a day to sustain good levels of circulating blood sugars. In fact it is better for your digestive system to eat smaller and more regular meals. I am sure you are all too aware of that awful heavy, bloated and full feeling after a big meal, so smaller meals at regular intervals are much better. That is how nature designed us and most mammals. Prehistoric man would have 'eaten on the hoof'. It is only in times of shortage that mammals will tend to eat big meals – to help insure against times of shortage.

Raising your blood sugar by means of diet ensures that pressure is taken off the liver and adrenal glands. The liver should be our back-up support to supply blood sugars and should release blood sugar if food has not been eaten or more energy is required.

The adrenal glands are there to provide an emergency supply of blood sugar for the 'flight or fight' response. But the adrenals will soon run out if not sustained properly and reserves maintained.

So you can see there is a balancing act between: diet – blood sugars – optimum liver function – detoxing via the liver – and healing. All these components of our system are inter-reliant to gain maximum benefits to health and well-being.

Endometriosis diet advice relating to your Fertility & pregnancy

(Some of this advice is still relevant for those who are not seeking pregnancy just yet)

This is a question I am often asked. I am not at liberty to give you detailed advice about your fertility – that should come from a fertility specialist. However I can give you basic common-sense advice about your diet as it relates to your health to improve your fertility.

Firstly, does endometriosis affect your fertility? Well confusingly the answer is Yes and No. The natural bio-chemical actions for fertility are still taking place – unless you are on hormone drugs. However, the physical damage caused by implants or adhesions or blocked fallopian tubes may reduce your fertility. I have always felt that natural treatments and diet can fix many aspects of endometriosis, but some of the physical damage that has already been done, that cannot be resolved by natural methods, will probably require surgical intervention to correct the physical damage that has already taken place. But what we are aiming to do here with the advice in this book – *is to stop this disease developing any further*.

However, I have known and experienced personally, that natural treatments CAN reduce/shrink the size of cysts, soften scar tissue, and certain supplements that contain proteolytic enzymes can 'eat up scar tissue' by the action they have on fibrin. Proteolytic enzymes (which are digestive enzymes) help to dissolved fibrin, and fibrin is one of the bodily by-products that make up scar tissue. There is more advice about this in the free 'A to Z of Diet & Nutrition Advice' mini e-book I have written, which you can find here:

http://www.endo-resolved.com/support-files/diet_nutrition_endometriosis.pdf - Look under 'P' for proteolytic enzymes. (This bit of advice is relevant TO ALL ENDO SUFFERERS.)

Diet for fertility

Two key nutrients for healthy fertility are *zinc and folic acid*. A deficiency of zinc plays an important role in infertility. Zinc helps cell division in the development of the foetus, while a lack of zinc can decrease the production of healthy eggs prior to conception. Zinc is the only mineral conclusively shown to increase fertility rates.

Folic acid aids in the growth of the foetus and also prevents neural tube defects. Aside from its effect on the developing foetal nervous system; folic acid deficiency can also lead to miscarriage as well. If you are attempting to get pregnant you should maintain consistent daily intake of folic acid 4mg/day. Folic acid can be found in leafy green vegetables, lentils, asparagus, papaya, and broccoli.

Supplements

High-quality multivitamins are an excellent way to ensure that a diet contains enough nutrients. Vitamins containing zinc, folic acid and B vitamins are crucial. Vitamin B6 is rich in folic acid, while Vitamin B12 helps to absorb it. Magnesium, vitamin B6 and vitamin E boost progesterone levels vital to protect the fertilised egg.

Eat fish rich in omega 3 oils - These are oily fish like mackerel, herring, trout, and salmon. Omega 3 will support your body in many ways as well as assist fertility.

An Unhealthy Diet – Or Foods to Avoid

Foods containing preservatives and other chemicals, such as artificial sweeteners, should be avoided because they affect blood sugar levels and hormonal balance. Foods high in fat should also not be consumed – but these are excluded from the endometriosis diet anyway.

Rhubarb is said to inhibit pregnancy as well as peas as they contain a natural contraceptive called xylohydroquinone. But you would need to eat a significant amount to really interfere with fertility.

Fish and mercury – Methyl-mercury in fish mainly comes from mercury in ocean sediment that is transformed into methyl-mercury by microorganisms. This organic form of mercury is absorbed by the tissues of fish through their gills as they swim and through their digestive tracts as they feed.

Some fish contain more mercury than others - Mercury levels differ from one species of fish to the next. This is due to factors such as type of fish, size, location, habitat, diet and age. Fish that are predatory (eat other fish) are large and at the top of the food chain, and so tend to contain more mercury. Pregnant women and women intending to become pregnant should avoid shark, marlin and swordfish – but I don't think these are on the average shopping list!. You may also want to limit the amount of tuna you eat. Fortunately - everyday favourites such as cod, haddock and plaice are not affected at all by this advice.

But we have talked earlier about needing to eat fish from unpolluted waters. If you are lucky enough to live in a part of the world with clean sea waters, then your fish supplies that are caught locally should be safer.

Fertility in relation to the endometriosis diet

The diet focussed for endometriosis is totally safe for those wishing to achieve pregnancy. Simply increase your intake of the supplements – especially zinc and folic acid – to increase your chances and boost your fertility. Eat sensibly – in other words eat a balanced diet to give your body the variety of nutrients in needs.

And finally, the proof that this diet is safe and supportive for improved fertility comes from feedback of past readers who have successfully achieved pregnancy to full term as well as reduce their endometriosis at the same time.

A Word of Warning about Soy

This topic is rather long, but I wanted to drive the message home to ensure you got the whole picture. My concern is based on the fact that so many people simply churn out advice – usually the first thing they read elsewhere, and then simply pass it on. I did LOTS of research on soy because I felt somehow 'uncomfortable' with it as a food and source of protein.

(Please note – this is the same advice that I have written up on the website at Endo-Resolved, but I felt it important to have this advice to hand for you to read)

I was demi-vegetarian when I had endometriosis – some chicken occasionally and fish. The thought of eating soy based protein never appealed to me – ever. Now that I have really looked into the topic of SOY I am glad I never got a 'liking' for it. Read on and you see what I mean .....

Testimonial about soy:

'Thank you for the in-depth discussion on the pitfalls of soy both in the Recipe book and on your website! My endometriosis wasn't a problem until I went vegetarian and started eating soy products at every meal (soybean sausages, hamburgers, milk, even tofu in tapioca pudding and other baked goods). Because the pain didn't hit all at once, and I fell off the almost all soy diet, I didn't catch my mistake in time. Now, however, I can control my endo pain by staying away from soy, dairy, and peanuts! My mother, a life-long soy eater, didn't believe me when I initially figured out the cause of my pain. Resources like yours helped her to understand why I had still been having pain after two laparoscopies and a hellish year on Lupron. It was my diet all along! Thank you again!

Melissa. USA

In recent years soy has emerged as a 'near perfect' food, with supporters claiming it can provide an ideal source of protein, lower cholesterol, protect against cancer and heart disease, reduce menopause symptoms, and prevent osteoporosis, among other things.

There are two isoflavones found in soy, genistein and daidzen, the same two isoflavones promoted by the soy industry for everything from menopause relief to cancer protection, were said to '**demonstrate toxicity in oestrogen sensitive tissues and in the thyroid**'. That last sentence is most relevant for women with endometriosis.

There are two 'camps' for the use of soy in food. There is the traditional, oriental use of soy in fermented soy products. These products are produced naturally and do not contain the same chemicals and toxins of the modern highly processed use of soy.

The modern approach to the use of soy has come by default, by finding a use of the soy bean by-products after the extraction of oil from the bean. There was so much soy bean residue that extensive multi-million dollar campaigning and advertising was used to promote this new 'wonder-protein'.

The history of soy-bean use

The soybean did not serve as a food in China until the discovery of fermentation techniques, sometime during the Chou Dynasty. The first soy foods were fermented products like tempeh, natto, miso and soy sauce.

At a later date, possibly in the 2nd century BC, Chinese scientists discovered that a purée of cooked soybeans could be precipitated with calcium sulphate or magnesium sulphate (plaster of Paris or

Epsom salts) to make a smooth, pale curd - tofu or bean curd. The use of fermented and precipitated soy products soon spread to other parts of the Orient, notably Japan and Indonesia.

The Chinese did not eat unfermented soybeans as they did other legumes such as lentils because the soy bean contains large quantities of natural toxins or "anti-nutrients".

How soy is processed today – read on and feel disgusted!

Production of soy protein products takes place in industrial factories where a slurry of soy beans is first mixed with an alkaline solution to remove fibre, then precipitated and separated using an acid wash and, finally, neutralised in an alkaline solution.

Acid washing in aluminium tanks leaches high levels of aluminium into the final product. The resultant curds are spray-dried at high temperatures to produce a high-protein powder. A final indignity to the original soybean is high-temperature; a high-pressure extrusion processing of soy protein isolate to produce textured vegetable protein (TVP). *Hmmm – that sounds delicious!!*

The high-temperature processing of Soy has the unfortunate side-effect of so 'de-naturing' the other proteins in soy that they are rendered largely ineffective. Nitrites, which are potent carcinogens, are formed during spray-drying, and a toxin called lysinoalanine is formed during alkaline processing. Numerous artificial flavourings, particularly MSG, are added to soy protein isolate and textured vegetable protein products to mask their strong "beany" taste and to impart the flavour of meat.

Soy is found in dozens and dozens of items: granola, vegetarian chilli, a vast sundry of imitation animal foods, pasta, most protein powders and "power" bars, soy milk, soy yoghurts, soy based cheeses, to name just a few.

After multi-million dollar figures spent on advertising and intense lobbying to the Food and Drug Administration (FDA), about 74 % of U.S. consumers now believe soy products are healthy.

Here is a quote about soy from the book 'What Your Doctor May Not Tell You about Premenopause' by Dr. John Lee, one of the pioneers in the use of Natural Progesterone Cream.

'Please be wary of all the hype around soy. Although it does contain compounds that can help balance your hormones, it is far from a magic hormone balance solution. Soy contains compounds that block the absorption of needed nutrients like zinc and will disable enzymes your body needs to access other nutrients. It directly blocks thyroid function and protein absorption. Many people are allergic to soy products, and women who are extremely sensitive to oestrogens of any kind may react negatively to them.

The traditional Asian processing methods used to make fermented soy products--tofu, tempeh, and miso—get rid of most of the toxins and make the beneficial phytochemicals more available in the body. Tofu and tempeh are a nearly complete protein and as such are an excellent alternative to meat in a balanced meal. Miso stirred into hot water with a strip of kombu or nori (seaweeds) makes a satisfying soup base or beverage. To offset the negative side of soy, Dr. David Zava recommends eating fermented soy products and tofu as the Asians do, with a protein such as fish and a rich mineral source such as the sea-weeds.

Soy milks and soy protein powders aren't in the same league as the fermented soy products, so use them sparingly. There's a good chance that the soybean toxins are more concentrated in these products, and they may do you more harm than good over the long haul.'

However, for endometriosis sufferers we need to go into this a bit deeper ....

Health Hazards of Soy

This is the type of information (especially on websites) where so many people simply do not research the subject properly; they basically pass on the usual/standard advice - to eat soy in place of meat.

1. High levels of phytic acid in soy reduce assimilation of calcium, magnesium, copper, iron and zinc. Phytic acid in soy is not neutralised by ordinary preparation methods such as soaking, sprouting and long, slow cooking. High phytate diets have caused growth problems in children.

2. Trypsin inhibitors in soy interfere with protein digestion and may cause pancreatic disorders. In test animals soy containing trypsin inhibitors caused stunted growth.

3. Soy phytoestrogens disrupt endocrine function and have the potential to cause infertility and to promote breast cancer in adult women.

4. Soy phytoestrogens are potent anti-thyroid agents that cause hypothyroidism and may cause thyroid cancer. In infants, consumption of soy formula has been linked to autoimmune thyroid disease.

5. Vitamin B12 analogues in soy are not absorbed and actually increase the body's requirement for B12.

6. Soy foods increase the body's requirement for vitamin D.

7. Fragile proteins are denatured during high temperature processing to make soy protein isolate and textured vegetable protein.

8. Processing of soy protein results in the formation of toxic lysinoalanine and highly carcinogenic nitrosamines – chemicals to you and me.

9. Free glutamic acid or MSG, a potent neurotoxin, is formed during soy food processing and additional amounts are added to many soy foods.

10. Soy foods contain high levels of aluminium which is toxic to the nervous system and the kidneys

11. The various negative effects of soy weaken the immune system.

Phytic acid and soy

Phytic acid is a part of the soy bean's makeup which is found in the husk of the bean – and also totally destroys the credibility of the manufacturers' claims that soy products are a good source of calcium and help prevent osteoporosis. Because soy contains more phytic acid than any other grain or pulse, and because phytic acid impairs absorption of most minerals, especially calcium, soy actually strips your body of calcium.

Although not a household word, phytic acid has been extensively studied; there are literally hundreds of articles on the effects of phytic acid in the current scientific literature. Scientists are in general agreement that grain - and legume-based diets high in phytates - contribute to widespread mineral deficiencies in third world countries.

The soybean has one of the highest phytate levels of any grain or legume that has been studied, and the phytates in soy are highly resistant to normal phytate-reducing techniques such as long, slow cooking. Only a long period of fermentation will significantly reduce the phytate content of soybeans.

As mentioned earlier, phytic acid has been highlighted by Dian Mills in her book *Endometriosis - Healing through Diet and Nutrition*, as being a particular compound that is found in wheat. She speculates that it is the phytic acid in wheat which aggravates the symptoms of Endometriosis. Phytic acid is found at higher levels in soy than it is in wheat, but many women who use a diet for endometriosis are substituting their dairy and protein intake with soy products. This will obviously negate the benefits of a targeted diet for Endometriosis.

GM crop

Most soybeans are grown on farms that use toxic pesticides and herbicides, and many are from genetically engineered plants. When you consider that **two-thirds of all manufactured food** products contain some form of soy, it becomes clear just how many Americans are consuming GM products, whose long-term effects are completely unknown.

PR and soy

The public relations machine extolling the virtues of soy has been global and relentless. It has to be - there are at least 100 million acres of soy under cultivation in the United States alone, much of it genetically engineered.

The Monsanto Corporation has 45 million acres of genetically modified soybeans growing in the United States. American law permits these crops to be mixed with a small amount of organic soybeans, and the resultant combination may then be labelled organic! Can you believe that!

It is not only the media who bear responsibility for helping the soy industry carry out this mass - manipulation and brainwashing of the public. Many health professionals are so busy, and probably totally unaware of the truth about Soy, that they are unable to counsel and advise their patients correctly regarding diet.

> "There is a distinct herd instinct among people who 'work in science' which makes it easy to believe whatever sounds plausible, if a lot of other people are saying it is true. Sometimes powerful economic interests help people to change their beliefs. For example, two of the biggest industries in the world, the oestrogen industry and the soy bean industry, spend vast amounts of money helping people to believe certain plausible-sounding things that help them sell their products." *From a soy advice website.*

You are going to come across many sources of advice and information about soy, which will extol the wonderful virtues of this protein substitute. This advice will probably come from the PR machine of the soy growers. Research this subject further for yourself.

And finally, tofu is made from soy protein and here is a video that explains why this product is not suitable in your diet: http://articles.mercola.com/sites/articles/archive/2008/09/18/what-s-so-bad-about-tofu.aspx

---

Many women who change their old diet for a diet to control endometriosis will often be replacing the dairy and protein foods and substituting them with soy products. As mentioned earlier, these will include soy milk, soy spreads, soy cheeses, soy based burgers and substitute meats, tofu and many other alternative soy products.

You need to avoid all modern soy based foods and food substitutes. The only safe soy foods are those that come from eastern traditions of fermented foods like *miso, tempeh and tamari*. These foods are safe enough for the healthy person, but for women with Endometriosis their consumption needs to be monitored because of the high levels of phytoestrogens – more on this later.

There are thousands of recipe books loaded with so-called healthy meat alternatives, and 9 times out of 10 this includes alternative soy based products. People will be of the belief that their meat free, dairy free diet is safe and healthy, when in fact the opposite is true.

Testimonial:

'Many thanks for the endo site and your recipe book full of good advice. I was particularly interested in the hype about soy and how to be aware of the so called "pretty advertising". I have followed your

wheat free, diary free, red meat free, caffeine free advice and hey presto 8-10 weeks later symptoms have improved. I no longer need anti-inflammatory drugs, the irritable bowel symptoms have all but disappeared and I feel more energized by eating organic fruits and veg, and taking vitamin C and D. I am now working on external estrogens and how to avoid them in household products and body products. Thanks Carolyn for all your hard work.' Val, USA

The list above covers the ingredients that are NOT in this book. Now let's look very briefly at some other basic changes that can help your diet and support healing....

The Good stuff!!!!

Oils

This includes the oils that you cook with, the oils you use in dressings, and the oils you will use in baking instead of dairy fats (margarine).

The types of oils you use on a diet for endometriosis are important.

Processed vegetable oils are bad for you. During the extraction process of many oils, they undergo a heat and/or chemical process to remove the oil from the seed and to clarify and deodorise it. This process completely changes the molecular structure and in turn the body will treat it as a harmful chemical. It then has to be eliminated from the body by the liver by manufacturing specific enzymes. If your body's metabolism is compromised in any way, like disease, this will cause further ill health.

The only vegetable oils to eat are those which have been produced by being cold-pressed during the processing.

You need to be using oils that metabolise into prostaglandin series one and three, because they are anti-inflammatory. (You will find a full explanation of Prostaglandins further on). Also, natural oil molecules are synthesised by the body to protect the cell membranes. This stops harmful chemicals entering and damaging the cells.

Ideally you need to be using **natural, unrefined cold-pressed oils**. They need to belong to the group of oils that contain essential fatty acids, like omega 6 and omega 3. These can be found in:

- Olive oil
- safflower oil
- walnut oil
- flax seed oil
- linseed oil
- borage oil
- star flower oil

Coconut Oil is great in your diet – I bet you thought the opposite was true

Coconut oil should be seriously considered to include in your diet and in some dishes you can cook with it to add a light coconut flavour – great in some soups for example.

The health benefits of Coconut oil appear to be far reaching, and some members of the press are calling this a 'wonder food'. The ability of Coconut oil to boost the immune system, as well as soothe and repair digestive disorders will be very relevant and supportive if you have Endometriosis along with digestive issues of any kind.

Coconut oil is now deemed as one of the healthiest oils you can consume. It is rich in lauric acid, which is known for being anti-viral, antibacterial and anti-fungal. You can even use it on your skin to help prevent wrinkles.

In addition to tasting and smelling great, the health benefits of Coconut oil include:

* Help you lose weight as it speeds up the metabolism
* Reduce your risk of heart disease
* Lower your cholesterol
* Improve conditions in those with diabetes and chronic fatigue
* Improve Crohn's, IBS, and other digestive disorders
* Prevent other disease and routine illness with its powerful antibacterial, anti-viral and anti-fungal agents
* Increase metabolism and promote healthy thyroid function
* Boost your daily energy
* Rejuvenate your skin and prevent wrinkles

There is a widespread misconception that coconut oil is bad for you because it contains saturated fat – again, this advice comes from only knowing half the facts. Fats are categorised as short, medium, or long-chain molecules depending on how many carbon molecules they contain. Close to two-thirds of the saturated fat in coconut oil is made up of medium-chain fatty acids, which have anti-microbial properties, are easily digested by the body for quick energy, and are beneficial to the immune system. Far from being dangerous, the saturated fat in coconut oil is actually health promoting.

Both coconut oil and coconut milk have great health benefits – but the oil contains more health benefits.

Uses for coconut milk you can try out and experiment with for yourself

* Stir fries, works great by simply adding some curry paste - works especially well in fish stir fries.
* On fruit - A couple of tablespoons coating some fresh cut up fruit is a wonderful breakfast or snack.
* Diluted with cereal as an alternative to dairy milk
* Mixed with mashed avocado to make a dip, perfect with some cut up veg like carrot
* Anywhere you would have previously used milk or cream.

There are various good books about coconut oil and milk which also include some helpful recipes – see back of book

Quality of Oil

You need be absolutely certain, however, of the *quality* and effectiveness of whatever coconut oil brand you choose. There is a very wide variety in terms of the types of coconuts, and the manufacturing processes used to make the oil.

Most commercial coconut oils are RBD (refined, bleached, and deodorised). RBD oils do contain the medium chain fatty acids; however they also contain chemicals used in processing. You need to purchase cold-pressed, virgin coconut oil - the same as you would for olive oil - to get the health benefits without the added chemicals.

Bad Press in the Past

In the past Coconut oil has got a bad press and a bad reputation in turn. Based on some flawed studies performed over four decades ago, some of which used primarily hydrogenated coconut oils, a powerful 'anti-saturated fat movement' began. Hydrogenated oils are oils with trans-fatty acids, which have been altered from their original chemical composition and have been shown to raise cholesterol levels and lead to heart disease and other health problems. You should not consume hydrogenated oils, whether it is coconut or another vegetable oil. Fortunately, the benefits of un-adulterated coconut oil are beginning to gain some positive media exposure, as researchers realise its health-promoting quality

How coconut oil helps health

Coconut oil's saturated fat is of the medium-chain fatty acid (MCFA) variety. These MCFAs are digested more easily and utilised differently by the body than other fats. Whereas other fats are stored in the body's cells, the MCFAs in coconut oil are sent directly to the liver where they are immediately converted into energy. So when you eat coconut oil, the body uses it immediately to make energy rather than store it as body fat. Because this quick and easy absorption puts less strain on the pancreas, liver and digestive system, coconut oil "heats up" the metabolic system and is an excellent support for the whole process of elimination and detox.

For those with Crohn's and IBS, the anti-inflammatory and healing effects of coconut oil have been shown to play a role in soothing inflammation and healing injury in the digestive tract. Interestingly, researchers have demonstrated the benefits of coconut oil on patients with digestive problems, including, Crohn's disease since the 1980s. Its anti-microbial properties also promote intestinal health by killing troublesome micro-organisms that may cause chronic inflammation.

Coconut oil supports the immune system by ridding the body of harmful micro-organisms, thus relieving stress on the body. With fewer harmful organisms taxing the body's energy, the immune system can function better.

For women with Endometriosis, this oil can be incorporated into your diet in many ways - as cooking oil, added to salads in a dressing, as a spread in place of butter, or added to your baking. And don't forget that you can use it straight on your skin as a moisturiser.

Tomatoes – help prevent scar tissue

Great news if you like tomatoes …..

A chemical in tomatoes called Lycopene has been found to help prevent scarring associated with endometriosis. A study found that when cells taken from the internal scar tissue were exposed to lycopene in the laboratory they reacted positively. This same chemical is also a powerful antioxidant which mops up other oxidative chemicals that cause damage in the body.

Lycopene was also found to prevent adhesions, where scar tissue builds up and can cause internal organs to stick together after surgery. From an article in The Daily Mail:

'Dr Tarek Dbouk, from Wayne State University in Detroit, Michigan, said lycopene could become a safe and cheap treatment in conditions such as endometriosis.

In a laboratory study, presented at the American Society for Reproductive Medicine conference in San Francisco, the nutrient was found to cut the presence of proteins that cause scar tissue to form by between 80% and 90%.

Simply increasing the amount of lycopene in the diet through taking supplements or increasing the intake of tomatoes could become a preventative treatment before abdominal surgery and may lead to new treatments for endometriosis, he said.

You can easily increase your intake of tomatoes with soups, pasta sauces, and tomatoes included in casserole mixes. Apparently lycopene is taken up by the body better when tomatoes are cooked as this alters its structure. Lycopene is also present in papaya and rosehips.

Fibre

Fibre plays a very important role in maintaining a healthy digestive system. Having a good fibre balance in your diet will help to alleviate constipation and will also help to flush excess oestrogens from the body. Also fibre binds the oestrogens and inhibits their re-absorption. The best source of dietary fibre is from whole foods, unrefined wholegrain cereals, nuts, seeds, berries and pulses. Fibrous vegetables like celery, carrot, potato and other root vegetables, legumes and linseed meal are also good sources of fibre.

Let's clear up any 'grey areas' regarding fibre and constipation!

There are two types of fibre – soluble and non-soluble – and you need to eat a balance of the two. The non-soluble fibre is found in the rough part of foods – the husks of grain, the skins of certain fruits and vegetables. The soluble fibre is found in higher amounts in fruit and vegetables as well as in legumes.

The words *soluble* or *non-soluble* refer to whether a fibre is dissolved and broken down in your system. If you eat mainly non-soluble fibre you could end up being MORE constipated because this type of fibre will *absorb water* from your gut as it goes through the digestive system – this action is supposed to support and aid digestion and stop constipation, and this is the advice many doctors will give.

However, absorbing water from your gut will slow down transit time as things dry up – and the slower this transit time takes the dryer your gut becomes – and this then becomes more difficult to get through your system to excrete as stools. On the other hand, if you eat lots of soluble fibre then you could end up with 'the runs'. So please balance your fibre between the two types to stop any issues of constipation developing. So many doctors simply say .. 'Are you getting enough fibre', without explaining that you need to eat a balance of the two types. If you stuff yourself with brown rice you will just clog yourself up!

Whole Grains for Fibre – the non-soluble fibre

What are whole grains anyway.....

Whole grains are foods that contain the entire kernel or grain, or the entire kernel that is edible. Some examples are oatmeal, whole cornmeal, popcorn, brown rice, whole rye, and barley, quinoa, and spelt. But spelt and rye is not included in the book here as they are both grains that are closely related to wheat.

When grains are refined, much of the nutritional value is lost by removing the kernel. Whole grains are more wholesome and you have a better chance of getting the vitamins, minerals, folic acid, magnesium, vitamin E, antioxidants, and other unknown factors that you lose when grains are refined.

Easy ways to add more whole grains:

You can easily add whole grains to your meals. Try some of the following:

*   Add half a cup of cooked bulgur, wild rice, or barley to stuffings for stuffed vegetables etc.
*   Add half a cup of cooked wild rice, brown rice, sorghum or barley to your favourite home-made soup.
*   Use whole corn-meal for corn cakes, corn breads and corn muffins.
*   Make risottos, pilaffs and other rice-like dishes with whole grains such as barley, brown rice, bulgur, millet, quinoa
*   Enjoy whole grain salads like tabbouleh (using wheat-free couscous which you can buy in health stores), rice salad, whole grain wheat-free pasta salads etc.
*   Look for cereals made with grains like kamut, kasha (buckwheat) or grano.

Fruit and Vegetables

You do need to peel or thoroughly was all your vegetables and fruit from commercial suppliers, as the skins will probably contain dioxins picked up from pesticides and sprays. There is no guarantee that organic fruit has not picked up some of these harmful chemicals. Some dishonest practises have been uncovered as far as imported 'organic' produce is concerned from overseas.

Unless the fruit and vegetables you purchase are local organic produce, it may well have been sprayed several times as it was growing and probably again whilst it was in storage. So the message is to peel and wash everything.

Eating Organic

If at all possible try to eat organic produce for your diet. This applies not only to your fruit and vegetables, but to other produce as well. There are an increasing number of food stores and supermarkets who are beginning to supply a wide range of organic produce. This can include organic rice, pulses, different flours, nuts, tinned foods, frozen foods - in fact most foods can be purchased these days that are organic. Many people think of shopping for organic food only for fresh produce like fruit, vegetables and meat, but today there are a lot of wholesome organic foods available.

OK, it may be more expensive to purchase organic foods, but you can make savings by not eating those expensive convenience foods. As the number of organic growers increases the cost of organic foods will continue to drop, and in summer you can easily grow your own salads.

If you are going to include meat in your diet, then this needs to come from an organic farm, where the live-stock has been raised and fed organically. But remember you need to exclude red meat from your diet.

Added to this, I advise you to try and purchase from local organic growers. As I have mentioned earlier, there have been some unscrupulous practises uncovered where growers/distributors who import their produce, which has been found to be far from organic because of the use of sprays and chemicals.

It stands to reason that any foods which are going to be put into storage and then shipped around the world will have to be treated in some way to stop it rotting. It does not bare thinking about. Some of your food may have even been gassed - especially if it going to be in storage for months while it is shipped. The bottom line - do try and purchase from your local growers, and you will be supporting local business as well and helping your local economy.

Eat foods in season

As well as food being cheaper if it is in season, it is also more suited to the climate for that time of year. Summer foods are generally juicy and lighter; winter foods are heavier and contain more carbohydrates which help to keep you warm in the winter.

Foods to aid excretion of oestrogens from the body

Foods containing natural plant sterols can be helpful in your diet. They are thought to block the oestrogenic receptors, so in turn excess oestrogen in the body cannot 'lock-in' to these receptors. These include:

- peas, beans and pulses
- red and purple berries
- garlic
- apples
- parsley
- fennel
- brassicas: cabbage, cauliflower etc.
- nuts and seeds
- celery, carrots
- rhubarb
- sage

Anti-yeast foods to assist dealing with Candida

I have not gone into great depths with advice about Candida. You can obtain that in other sources. But the advice throughout this book and the recipes it contains will stand you in good stead if you do have a Candida overgrowth.

What is Candida - Candida albicans is a yeast like organism that lives naturally in small amounts in your mouth, gastrointestinal tract and skin. The body's natural defence against fungal and yeast infections is the production of friendly bacterial flora that keeps it in check.

Candida is controlled by a properly functioning immune system and "friendly" bacteria. However, if the number of friendly bacteria is decreased, the immune system is weakened or other conditions for yeast proliferation occur. Candida albicans may shift from a yeast to a fungal form and start to invade the body and cause a multitude of health problems.

Donna Gates, in her book, "The Body Ecology Diet: Recovering Your Health and Rebuilding Your Immunity" has shown strong connection between endometriosis and candida yeast overgrowth. A study by the Woman's Hospital of Texas examined 50 women with endometriosis and found that 40 women showed bacterial overgrowth. After eight weeks following the candida/endometriosis diet, significant reduction in symptoms was achieved.

Foods that assist with cleansing the body of Candida include garlic, onions, cabbage, broccoli, watercress, mustard cress, cauliflower, turnips, and cinnamon. Aloe Vera juice and pau d'arco tea are also very useful for this purpose.

Bromelain to aid pain and inflammation

The enzyme Bromelain from the stem of the pineapple is effective in inhibiting the inflammatory prostaglandins. In an extensive five-year study of more than 200 people experiencing inflammation as a result of surgery, traumatic injuries, wounds and pain, 75 % of the study participants had good to excellent improvement with Bromelain. Most of the people in this study were discharged from the hospital in only eight days—half the usual amount of time.

Try adding additional pineapple to your diet to see what effect it has on your symptoms of endometriosis. You can easily add pineapple chunks to the top of pizza (wheat-free), in puddings, eaten by itself, or juiced.

Noni juice

The Noni fruit is a natural tropical fruit found to contain over 150 beneficial components which include 20 amino acids, 9 of which are essential because they are not produced in the body. Noni also includes vitamin A, all the B vitamins, vitamin C, vitamin E, beta carotene, linoleic acid, bromelain, pectin, calcium, magnesium and zinc.

At present noni is known to be the best source of bromelain, as it contains 40 times more than any other known food, including pineapple.

It is a more expensive option than pineapple, but the added health benefits are worth the price. There are a few testimonials I have found from women with endometriosis who have used noni juice and have found that their health has greatly improved and some women have seen complete elimination of the symptoms of endometriosis by using noni. As with all natural remedies, you need to use the juice for a few months before you really begin to notice the changes or improvements in your health.

Green Tea

There are many health benefits to be gained by consuming green tea. There is one health benefit in particular which will be very appropriate for women with endometriosis, and that is the **ability of green tea to protect the body at a molecular level from the toxic effects of Dioxins.**

The fact that researchers are discovering that green tea can protect the body from the damaging effects of dioxins is valuable advice for women with endometriosis, given that many researchers feel that dioxins could be the cause of endometriosis.

Green tea is actually the same plant as its more well-known cousin black tea; however, special processing retains a far greater antioxidant profile in green tea leaves, resulting in a far more superior beverage for supporting health. Numerous scientific studies now document the tremendous benefits of drinking green tea.

A study by researchers at Rochester University suggesting that green tea's ability to fight cancer is even more potent and varied than scientists had initially known about. The researchers found chemicals in green tea that shut down a key molecule that can play a role in the development of cancer. The molecule - the aryl hydrocarbon receptor, or AH - can activate genes in a harmful way. Dioxins and tobacco smoke cause the molecule to trigger potentially harmful gene activity. Two chemicals in green tea - similar to the anti-cancer flavonoids in cabbage, broccoli, grapes, and red wine - inhibit AH activity.

There are numerous chemical contaminants which enter the body and cause their damaging effects through the molecular pathway. This same pathway is shut down by the active ingredients in green tea. These chemicals include dioxins, some PCB's and other chemicals that are far too complex to need mentioning.

Drink de-caffeinated Green Tea

It is well known that caffeine aggravates the symptoms of Endometriosis, and fortunately you can purchase decaffeinated green tea. An average cup (6 oz) of green tea contains approximately 30 milligrams of caffeine. This compares to a cup of black tea, which has about 40 milligrams, and a cup of brewed coffee, which has 120 milligrams of caffeine.

A cup of naturally **decaffeinated** green tea contains only 2 milligrams of caffeine per cup, so this will be safe to drink.

The effect of the decaffeination process on the health benefits of green tea depends on which process is used. A natural decaffeination process preserves the antioxidants found in green tea by using only spring water and effervescence (CO_2 method) to take the caffeine out. Some green tea brands use the chemical, ethyl acetate, which can destroy most of the best antioxidants found in green tea. A double negative of more unwanted chemicals plus the health benefits of the tea being removed.

If you are to drink green tea then purchase naturally decaffeinated organic green tea, which will not upset or aggravate your symptoms of Endometriosis. Some people find that this tea does have rather a bitter taste, but I have found new products with different fruits or vanilla added to give flavouring and sweetness.

Supplement for a healthy intestinal flora

Our intestinal flora should have a natural balance of friendly bacteria which undertake a variety of vital tasks for our health.

With long term use of antibiotics or hormones these friendly bacteria can be destroyed. As mentioned earlier, this is one of the possible causes of Candida and other digestive problems.

You can replace this healthy intestinal flora by supplementing with Lactobacillus acidophilus, which is available at most health food stores. You will not need to take it continuously - only as long as it takes to restore the intestinal flora in your gut. This should only take a few months on average.

This friendly bacterium is also found in natural 'live' yoghurt – discussed earlier. Adding 'live' yoghurt to your diet may not be sufficient to rebalance the 'friendly' bacteria, so a supplement to reintroduce this bacterium is advised.

Lactobacillus acidophilus provides a variety of potential health benefits. These include:

- Replacing the friendly intestinal bacteria destroyed by broad-spectrum antibiotics - these bacteria aid digestion and help suppress disease-causing bacteria
- Reducing the recurrence rate of lower urinary tract infections and cystitis (bladder inflammation)
- Improving lactose absorption in people with lactose intolerance
- Preventing recurring vaginal infections
- Possibly enhancing immune functions in immune compromised individuals
- Aiding the production of some B vitamins and vitamin K, and aiding in the breakdown of food
- Alleviating symptoms of irritable bowel syndrome and address candida
- I have also found that a higher dose can help to address problems of constipation

Dietary supplements

There are various references to individual dietary supplements woven throughout the book. The following is a list of supplements that will help women with Endometriosis to support various bodily processes:

Magnesium - is a mineral and is believed to ease cramping with menstruation. It also assists with maintaining water levels in the gut and can help with the problem of constipation

Zinc - is essential for enzyme activity, helping cells to reproduce which will help with healing. Zinc is also reported to boost the immune system and helping to create an emotional sense of well-being. Also vital to improve fertility.

Calcium - levels of calcium in menstruating women decrease 10 to 14 days before the onset of menstruation. Deficiency may lead to muscle cramps, headache or pelvic pain.

Iron - women with endometriosis tend to have very heavy periods which can lead to an iron deficiency. This can lead to anaemia which is characterized by extreme fatigue and weakness.

B vitamins - these are important for the breakdown of proteins, carbohydrates and fats in the body. B vitamins are reported to improve the emotional symptoms of endometriosis, and have proved helpful in dealing with PMT

Vitamin C - is well known for helping to boost the immune system and help provide resistance to disease. It is also used in the body to build and maintain collagen within the body.

Vitamin A - is another immune system booster

Vitamin E - plays an important role by increasing oxygen carrying capacities and also strengthens the immune system

Selenium - when taken together with vitamin E has been reported to decrease inflammation associated with Endometriosis, as well as immune system booster.

There is additional advice to be found about vitamins, minerals and dietary supplements in the free mini e-book 'A to Z Glossary of Diet and Nutrition' You can download the e-book direct from here: http://www.endo-resolved.com/support-files/diet_nutrition_endometriosis.pdf

A good quality multi-vitamin supplement is a good way to cover all bases, and you can add other specific supplements to target you own health requirements. Evening Primrose Oil, a good quality probiotic plus a proteolytic enzyme like serrapeptase are excellent additional supplements to take and the three that I would choose to go with a multi-vitamin.

Water - the food of life

When it comes to regeneration and rejuvenating the body, water is the most important nutrient of all. When you become dehydrated the chemical reactions in your cells become sluggish. Also your body cannot build new tissue effectively, toxic products build up in your blood-stream, your blood volume decreases and less oxygen and fewer nutrients are transported to your cells. Dehydration also makes you feel weak and tired and unable to concentrate.

The brain is seventy-five per cent water, this is why the quantity and quality of water you drink also affects how you feel and think. For mental clarity and emotional balance you need plenty of water. Drinking enough also provides us with energy; it stops us from having water-retention because the body is not in a state of panic and holding onto water all the time; in turn, water assists with banishing cellulite.

So you can see the vital importance of water for our bodies to stay in balance. The quality of water you drink matters a lot. You can either buy quality spring water or get yourself a good water filter and use it always, changing the filter regularly. Bottled waters differ tremendously. Some of those sold in plastic containers in the super-market are nothing more than tap water which has been run through conditioning filters to remove the taste, while doing nothing to improve the quality.

For basic good health, you need to be drinking around eight big glasses of water a day. Getting into the water habit will quench your appetite, heighten your energy levels, improve the look of your skin, as well as provide all those health benefits.

Meat

Yes you can eat white meat, but it will need to be organically reared and fed, and you should ideally only eat chicken or turkey - remember the issue with red meats and prostaglandins that cause inflammation. You do not need me to tell you how to cook your favourite recipes for chicken, so I have not included any here. Use the ideas included in the book of other ingredients to include, so you can adapt any of your favourite dishes.

Fish

Fish is fine for the endometriosis diet, and the fish which are of most benefit are the ones that contain beneficial fish oils that help to reduce inflammation. These include herring, mackerel, sardines, pilchards, salmon, trout and tuna.

What you **do** need to be careful about is eating fish that comes from clean water sources free from pesticides and dioxins. But how do we know where our fish is coming from. Even the fishermen will not know if their stock is from polluted or unpolluted waters.

It is safer to eat fish that has come from the sea, from <u>deep</u> waters where pollution is less. However, most of the fish from the list above are **not** deep water fish. The best way around this is to go to specialist fish farms, where you can purchase salmon or trout. Even better, you can search out these fish farms where they raise the stock organically.

Salt

We need salt in our diets. If we had a salt free diet we would need to take iodine supplements. A lot of table salt is actually iodized these days with additives. One of the key functions of iodine is to maintain the health of the thyroid. There are many women with endometriosis who appear to have imbalances of their thyroid gland. In turn, one of the functions of the thyroid is to control the hormone balances in the body.

Common table salt is extracted from rock salt as brine, and then re-crystallised. There is no goodness in this form of salt. Sea salt, on the other hand provides us with natural iodine as well as other minerals.

Where the recipes in this book suggest the use of salt, please use sea salt so that you can make use of the natural minerals that you need.

Bodily Chemicals and Hormones - the science bit!

Prostaglandins

This is the only really scientific subject we will cover, but it is worth you getting to understand the important role that prostaglandins have to play.

Prostaglandins are very relevant for women with Endometriosis because of the critical reaction and inter-action between endometrial tissue, digestive enzymes, pain and inflammation and various prostaglandin activities.

What you eat will directly affect the levels of different Prostaglandins produced by your body. There are good prostaglandins and bad prostaglandins. It's no wonder we can get confused!

Functions of Prostaglandins - some basics

Prostaglandins have a variety of physiological effects on the body including:

- Activation of the inflammatory responses at the sites of damaged tissue, and production of pain and fever. When tissues are damaged, white blood cells flood the site to try to minimise tissue destruction. Prostaglandins are produced as a result.
- Blood clots form when a blood vessel is damaged. A type of prostaglandin called thromboxane stimulates constriction and clotting of platelets. Also the opposite happens and prostaglandin 12 (PG12) is produced on the walls of blood vessels where clots should not be forming. (The body is very, very clever. It knows what to do, where to do it and when.)
- Certain prostaglandins are involved with the introduction of labour and other reproductive processes, and the role of fertility. PGE2 causes uterine contractions and has been used to induce labour.
- Prostaglandins are involved in several other organs and systems such as the gastrointestinal tract, cell growth and the immune system response.

Chemical Messengers

Prostaglandins vary somewhat from one another based upon subtle differences in their chemical structures. These small variations are believed to be responsible for the immense diversity of effects they have on the body. In general, prostaglandins act in a manner similar to that of hormones, by stimulating target cells into action. However, they differ from hormones in that they act locally, near their site of synthesis, and they are metabolised very rapidly. Interestingly, the same prostaglandins act differently in different tissue. (The in-built intelligence of the human body, which we will never understand)!

Prostaglandins in bite sizes! – The science bit !

This is a brief but detailed description of prostaglandins and you may want to come back to this later – it gets a bit complex!! It took me weeks to get to grips with this subject and understand all the complexities. I just hope I have written it up for you to be able to follow.

- Prostaglandins are chemical mediators, or 'local' hormones. Whereas hormones circulate in the blood stream to influence distant tissues, prostaglandins act locally on adjacent cells
- Prostaglandins serve as a catalyst for a large number of processes including the movement of

calcium and other substances into and out of cells, dilation and contraction, inhibition and promotion of blood clotting, regulation of secretions including digestive juices and hormones, control of fertility, cell division and growth

- Prostaglandins are produced in the cells by the action of enzymes on essential fatty-acids
- From the discoveries to date of the number and complexity of prostaglandins, they have been divided into 'Series' type prostaglandins. Most commonly known to women with endometriosis are the prostaglandin Series 1 and Series 2 for their opposing effects or cause on pain messengers and inflammation
- In simple terms, the Series 2 prostaglandins play a role in swelling and inflammation at sites of damage or injury. They also play a role in inducing birth, in regulating temperature, lowering blood pressure, and in the regulation of platelet forming and clotting. The role of Series 2 Prostaglandins does serve a vital role for the body for without it you would bleed to death from the slightest cut. However, in excess, these prostaglandins are harmful and many diseases are directly linked to excessive inflammation and blood clotting
- Series 1 prostaglandins have the opposite effect of the Series 2 prostaglandins. Series 1 reduce inflammation, dilate blood vessels, and inhibit blood clotting. The strong anti-inflammatory properties help the body recover from injury by reducing pain and swelling.
- No doubt this is a simplistic definition of the role of these different substances, which will be more complex and subtle, but research is still being done into how prostaglandins work.
- More recent research has focused on the balance between Series 2 and another group, the Series 3 prostaglandins. The Series 2 group is involved in intense actions, often in response to some emergency such as injury or stress. The Series 3 group has a modulating effect.
- The Series 3 prostaglandins are formed at a slower rate and work to deal with excessive Series 2 prostaglandin production.
- **Negative prostaglandins** - Many of you will have heard the term 'Antagonistic Prostaglandins' - in simple terms this means unfriendly prostaglandins – the sequence of 'events' and production of unfriendly prostaglandins through the food chain goes like this:
- *Antagonistic prostaglandins* are made from a fatty acid called *arachidonic acid* (I can't help thinking of spiders when that term is used - arachnid being the generic term for spiders, but this word seems relevant as spiders and other arachnids like scorpions are classed as '8 legged aggressive predators'. The same can be said of the predatory nature of antagonistic prostaglandins.)
- *Arachidonic acid* is obtained from animal products - meat and dairy
- Arachidonic acid can also be made from another fatty acid called *linoleic acid*, through the animal food chain consumption
- *Linoleic acid* is a fatty acid found in plant oils, such as corn oil, soybean oil, and other light vegetable oils. We also obtain linoleic acid from meat and dairy products (because the animals eat plants and store Linoleic acid)
- **Beneficial prostaglandins** - are made from a fatty acid found mostly in marine plants and fish known as EPA (eicosapentaenoic acid)
- EPA is the most important member of an exclusive group of three fatty acids called the "omega-3 fatty acids"
- This group includes alpha linoleic acid (ALA), eicosapentaenoic acid (EPA), and docosahexaenoic acid (DHA)
- ALA is made in the chloroplasts of green plants from linoleic acid. In mammals, linoleic acid is converted to arachidonic acid that is used to make the antagonistic prostaglandins. BUT, in the green plant the same linoleic acid is converted into the beneficial ALA
- ALA is important because it serves as the building material for EPA
- EPA is the most critical of the omega 3 fatty acids. It is the only material that our bodies use to make the beneficial prostaglandins that help reduce inflammation
- DHA is another omega 3 fatty acid. It is an integral part of eye and brain tissue. It is made by marine algae, plankton, fish and mammals from EPA. Fish accumulate DHA in their oily tissue, along with EPA
- It is now known that an excess of oleic acid (found chiefly in olive oil and nuts), known as the essential fatty acid group (EFA), will inhibit the prostaglandin pathway. But the block being set up is one which will inhibit the Series 2 prostaglandins - the ones which cause inflammation and

swelling. This is why women with endometriosis are advised to change the oil in their diet to only include the oils which will block Series 2. Evening Primrose Oil, Fish Oils, Flax seed oil, and Borage oil, which contain omega-3 fatty acids are also used by women with endometriosis to help shift the balance of prostaglandins and reduce the inflammatory action caused by Series 2 prostaglandins

- Aspirin, a non-steroidal anti-inflammatory, was discovered over 100 years ago. It works by blocking prostaglandins that are produced in inflamed or injured tissues and cause the sensation of pain. It also acts centrally: the salicylate and acetate parts of aspirin's chemical structure (aspirin is acetyl salicylic acid) cross separately into the brain and spinal cord. There they act on prostaglandins in sites in the central nervous system known to be involved in both the perception and transmission of pain.

- Prostaglandins are released by the endometrium during the menstrual cycle. Some women release more prostaglandin during menstruation than others. These higher levels of prostaglandins in women with severe dysmenorrhoea (painful periods) results in increased uterine contractions and muscular spasm.

Prostaglandins and pain messengers

Prostaglandins serve a variety of regulatory functions within the body. One of these functions is to assist the transmission of pain signals to the brain so that you are readily alerted that damage or dysfunction has occurred within the body.

When damage occurs to the body, certain prostaglandins are formed from the unsaturated fatty acids released by damaged cells. The production of a particular group of prostaglandins amplifies the amount of pain experienced by serving as a pain activator. They increase the sensitivity of the nerves to pain impulses. By reducing the synthesis of prostaglandins, the amount of pain stimuli sent to the brain is correspondingly reduced. This is usually achieved by the use of aspirin which blocks the production of pain messenger prostaglandins.

Alternatively, by making changes in your diet you can shift the prostaglandin production from the negative inflammatory prostaglandins to the anti-inflammatory prostaglandins.

Prostaglandins and inflammation

Prostaglandins are known as local hormones - they are released from cells and bring about changes in neighbouring cells that carry specific prostaglandin receptors in their membranes. The influence which prostaglandins have depends upon the type of tissue they are acting upon.

Such action may be direct, or as a result of modifying the actions of other signalling molecules. As well as signalling and influencing pain messengers to the brain, prostaglandins will interact with other chemicals in the body when there is damage. They will also intensify the effects of other chemical mediators such as histamine.

Acting in concert these substances can bring about vasodilatation (widening of blood vessels) and an increase in the permeability of capillaries supplying the damaged area, encouraging the migration of phagocytes (cells that remove unwanted substances). Phagocytes are white blood cells - that engulf invading micro-organisms, and then kill them. They are part of our natural defence against infection from the blood through capillary walls into the damaged tissue. As a result of these changes, the blood supply to the area increases, the tissues swell, causing inflammation and pain subsequently occurs.

Prostaglandins and Diet

You should have gathered by now that the KEY way to shift the production of prostaglandins - from the negative (inflammatory / pain messenger / womb contracting type) to the positive (anti-inflammatory / suppressing womb contractions and pain messenger type) - is through your diet, and most crucially by the types of fats and oils you include in your diet.

Several enzymes take part in the process that transforms fats into prostaglandins. These enzymes act as gatekeepers, channelling fats into the making of different prostaglandins. Like other enzymes in the body, they require specific nutrient coenzymes to do their job.

The enzyme delta-6-desaturase acts on linoleic acid - from most vegetable, nut and seed oils - to transform it to gamma-linoleic acid (GLA). GLA is used to make the anti-inflammatory series 1 prostaglandins and also supports healthy nervous system function.

The activity of delta-6-desaturase is affected by dietary factors. Trans-fatty acids from hydrogenated oils, too much saturated fat (found in meats, fried foods, junk foods and dairy products) in the diet, high stress, too much sugar or refined flours in the diet all slow down this enzyme down.

Vitamins and minerals you need to ensure good Prostaglandin production

The B vitamins are crucial for the conversion of linoleic acid to GLA, which is necessary to produce beneficial prostaglandins. Linoleic acid is an essential fatty acid (EFA), and it is found in foods such as fresh nuts and seeds, safflower oil, and Evening Primrose Oil.

The B vitamins are required to convert this essential oil into a form that can be used by the body to produce the good prostaglandins. The other vitamins and minerals you need are zinc, magnesium, vitamin C and calcium.

Summary

There are 2 groups of prostaglandins which are most relevant to endometriosis - Good or Bad.

Good - take part in the normal functions of the body without contributing to the processes which cause the negative effects of endometriosis

Bad - take part in the functions of the body which contribute to endometriosis symptoms and its negative effects i.e. pain, inflammation, digestive disturbance, connective tissue damage.

The way your body produces different types of prostaglandins can be controlled by what you include in your diet by consumption of different oils and foods. Some foods and oils will promote the negative prostaglandins because of subtle chemical reactions. In turn, other foods and oils will block that chemical reaction and stop the negative prostaglandins from being produced.

These potent chemicals act at an atomic level and are not always present in the body. They are produced in reaction to a sudden change or shock or injury in the body. Our bodies will produce them to act as warning signals, or to provide support to damaged tissue. The dual roles of prostaglandin Series 1 and 2 seem to be contradictory, but we obviously need both types of prostaglandins for the repair, maintenance and survival of the body.

If we did not suffer pain then we would not be alerted to the problem of damage within the body. Suffering pain is distressing, but in turn it is also telling us that something is wrong. It is fortunate that we now know how these particular prostaglandins work (be it in simple terms), so that women with endometriosis are able to alter the balance of prostaglandin production to reduce their symptoms by reducing the Series 2 prostaglandins, and aim to increase the Series 1 prostaglandins through their diet and with supplements.

To summarise what you need to eat to produce
the good prostaglandins:

- Olive oil, oily fish, nuts, seeds, cold-pressed vegetable oils, nut oils, sea food like seaweed
- Supplements of Evening Primrose Oil, Borage Oil, Fish oils, Starflower oil, Linseed oil

That's enough of the 'chemistry lesson' - but I am sure you can appreciate why I have included a sizeable amount of information of this topic. It could be that prostaglandins are the root cause of a lot of the pain of endometriosis. Being aware and better informed about this will ensure that you can adjust your diet accordingly and protect yourself from the bad prostaglandins and in turn reduce the amount of pain you feel.

Oestrogens and your diet for Endometriosis

Let's try and clarify, what I know is a complex and sometimes confusing subject - oestrogen and food intake!

OK let's start with all the different sources of oestrogen first, and then we know which is which, and where they come from. These are the ones I have learnt about in my research - there could be more that scientists have not found yet – yes that is possible, God forbid! - But the list goes like this:

Oestrogens - which are naturally made in the body?

Oestrogens are primarily made in the female ovaries and the male testes in humans and other animals. Known as the female hormones, oestrogens are found in greater amounts in females than males. These essential molecules influence growth, development and behaviour (puberty), regulate reproductive cycles (menstruation, pregnancy) and affect many other body parts (bones, skin, arteries, the brain).

Estrodiol is the most abundant and potent oestrogen hormone. Estrone and estriol are other types of oestrogens.

Oestrogen is commonly defined as "any of a family of steroid hormones that regulate and sustain female sexual development and reproductive function".

Xeno-estrogens - which are chemically based compounds that enter the body and can act like or interfere with the body's own oestrogen hormones. Most xeno-estrogens enter the body via the food chain with the use of herbicides, pesticides, industrial pollution washing onto pasture land and then consumed by live-stock, and the most widespread toxin on the planet - Dioxin - which mimics the action of oestrogen. These xeno-estrogens are also produced by chemicals found in toiletries.

Phytoestrogens - are plant based compounds that act like oestrogen in the body and are found in many foods we eat.

Many different plants produce compounds that may mimic or interact with oestrogen hormones. At least 20 compounds have been identified in at least 300 plants from more than 16 different plant families. Referred to as Phytoestrogens, these compounds are weaker than natural oestrogens and are found in herbs, grains (soybeans, wheat, and rice), vegetables (beans, carrots, and potatoes), fruits (dates, pomegranates, cherries, apples) and drink (coffee).

Most of us are exposed to many of these natural compounds through food. The two most studied groups of phytoestrogens are the lignans (compounds found in whole grains, fibres, flax seeds, and many fruit and vegetables) and the isoflavones (found in soybeans and other legumes). Because scientists have found phytoestrogens in human urine and blood samples, we know that these compounds can be absorbed into our bodies.

Phytoestrogens differ a great deal from synthetic environmental Xeno-estrogens, in that they are easily broken down, are not stored in tissue and spend very little time in the body.

There are differing opinions about phytoestrogens' role in health. When consumed as part of an ordinary diet, phytoestrogens are probably safe and may even be beneficial. In fact, some studies on cancer incidences in different countries suggest that phytoestrogens may help to protect against certain cancers (breast, uterus, and prostate) in humans.

On the other hand, eating very high levels of some phytoestrogens may pose some health risks. Reproductive problems have been documented in laboratory animals, farm animals and wildlife that ate very high (up to 100% of their diet) amounts of phytoestrogen-rich plants.

Even though humans almost never eat an exclusive diet of phytoestrogen-rich foods (even vegetarians), those who consume a diet that does contain a lot of soy are exposing themselves to health risks. As mentioned earlier in the topic of soy, there is a lot of soy protein added to every-day convenience foods.

Phytoestrogens behave like hormones, and like hormones, too much or too little can alter hormone-dependent tissue function. For this reason, women with endometriosis need to adjust their diet so as not to include too many phytoestrogen rich foods.

Endometriosis and Oestrogen

Endometriosis is activated and fed by oestrogen - this is well understood and documented. Women with endometriosis need to get their levels of oestrogen to a natural balance along with Progesterone and other hormones produced in the body.

Hormones are very powerful substances. It takes only microscopic amounts of any given hormone to activate a host of changes in the body.

It seems like an uphill battle to get the oestrogen levels back into balance for women with endometriosis. Even men are being affected by the amount of oestrogen in the environment. There are lower sperm counts and fertility problems. Children are beginning to enter puberty too early because of the oestrogen in the environment. Wildlife is being affected by the oestrogens in the environment.

The way to protect yourself and try and balance your hormones is to:

- Avoid all foods that have been polluted and contain compounds (xeno-estrogens) that act like oestrogens in your body. These compounds are stored in body fat so will not be excreted out of your system.
- Avoid toiletries that contain chemicals that mimic oestrogen for the same reason(If you want to know more about this topic please read this article here: http://www.endo-resolved.com/toiletries.html - which gives you advice about how to avoid toxic toiletries).
- Include in your diet the foods that contain phytoestrogens - **but this must be done in a balanced way** as mentioned earlier. The aim here is to take in phytoestrogens so that they block the pathways and stop your body absorbing xeno-estrogens. If you eat too many foods containing phytoestrogens then you are defeating the object - you will end up with too much oestrogen. It is all about balance. But remember, phytoestrogens pose less of threat to the body as they are much weaker and are not stored in the body.

Economics

When you have a diet that is reliant on freshly prepared foods, and you give up on all convenience foods (mostly), it can seem rather costly on finances and time.

Try shopping at your local market rather than at Supermarkets. In the UK we have weekly farmers markets where produce can be purchased direct from the grower – our local market trader will turn up in his van and sell all his produce in a matter of hours, as his food is much cheaper and not packaged in polystyrene trays and plastic.

For ingredients like nuts, seeds and pulses, see if there is a ware-house of whole-food co-op for whole-foods near you and buy in bulk.

Choose fruits and vegetables that are in season. They will be cheaper for obvious reasons. You could also try growing your own produce. You do not need a large vegetable plot to grow food. Many vegetables will grow quite happily in pots as long as you feed them regularly but they will need watering every day. My own freezer is loaded with green beans from this summer which were grown in a large pot on the patio. And you can't beat home-grown tomatoes for flavour and nutrition.

Is this labour intensive!

Here are some tips to help!

This is what I do to save time and effort - I have a large pan - about 16 inches across, with 2 handles so I can pick it up easier - my cauldron I call it, and I cook in bulk. I prepare enough of any given dish to eat one meal on the day it is cooked; one meal is put into a tub in the refrigerator (fridge to us Brits!) for another day, and put another lot into another tub and put in the freezer for another day.

Tip - the portion to go into the freezer - take this out of the cooking pan when the food is about three quarters cooked. This is because the freezing process tends to continue 'cooking' food and causes it to break down. So do not put fully cooked food in the freezer as it will thaw out a bit mushy, especially if it's a veg based dish.

Food preparation

I have given you a few tips above about saving time for food preparation. I need to advise you of some basic, and some labour saving equipment you are advised to have, otherwise you will find it a chore to prepare some of the delicious recipes. Many recipes here require the need to do a lot of blending of ingredients or to pulverise and break down raw ingredients into a puree. When you read the recipes this will be self-explanatory.

To do this you really need a food processor or heavy duty blender. It will be a good investment and you will find many uses for such kitchen equipment. (I even use mine to produce paper pulp when I'm making hand-made paper for my art-work!) If you purchase the better quality ones, they will work harder and last longer. Try to purchase a blender or food processor with a decent sized electric motor, as they will be able to work more efficiently.

There are many varieties on the market but it depends which country you live in as to which models are the best buy. If finances are a problem then consider asking your family for one as a Xmas or Birthday present.

Your Ideal Dietary Plan

- All fruit and veg to be fresh and organic if possible, and thoroughly washed/peeled before preparation
- Make sure your diet is balanced and interesting – you'll stick to the diet better if you enjoy your food
- I am a realist and if you are to eat any convenience foods/ready meals and sauces etc., always read the labels and do not buy foods with e-numbers and additives. You will get better quality convenience foods from health food stores – yes they do sell them, usually in the freezer or chill cabinet
- Avoid all foods that increase the bad prostaglandin production - especially red meat and dairy foods
- Eat all those foods that boost your immune system

Foods to Completely Avoid – a reminder:

- Sugar - in whatever form
- Red Meat
- Processed salt and high-salt products such as bouillon
- Dairy produce including all milk, cheese etc. – beware of sodium caseinate or whey in some packaged foods – try and keep packaged foods to a minimum
- Wheat and rye – and gluten if you feel you have gluten problems – this is becoming easier to do these days as many small, specialist food production companies are making gluten free flours and cake mixes
- Tea, coffee, fizzy drinks and alcohol – anything with caffeine
- Margarine and hydrogenated fats
- Soy milks/yoghurts and manufactured soy products; tofu, miso and tamari may be used in small amounts
- Tinned and packaged foods – my realistic exception to this is certain items like organic tinned tomatoes, coconut milks, organic non-sugar/salt added ready cooked beans/pulses
- Manufactured meat products, sausages, burgers, etc.
- Aspartame, saccharine, monosodium glutamate, food additives, chemicals, preservatives, nitrites, etc.

Eat more:

- Whole grains, (excluding wheat and rye), e.g. brown rice, millet, quinoa –   this will give you extra fibre that will help to remove excess oestrogens
- A balance of both types of fire – soluble and non-soluble
- Peas, beans and pulses
- Seeds and nuts
- Sprouted seeds – increases nutritional value tremendously
- Vegetables and salads – in whatever form
- Fruit – raw, lightly cooked, pureed for puddings and smoothies
- Oily Fish - if unsure about safety of fish then eat fish purchased from organically raised fish farms
- Tomatoes – great at reducing scar tissue
- Coconut oil and coconut milk - huge health benefits
- Drink green tea to help eliminate toxins and protect your system

Foods with a beneficial effect on the immune system

- Coconut Oil
- Onions
- Green tea
- Garlic (raw or lightly cooked)
- Pineapple (contains bromelain which is anti-inflammatory)
- Carrots (contain beta-carotene)
- Live yoghurt (to obtain healthy bacteria)
- Seeds: sesame, pumpkin etc.
- Sprouted seed - increases nutritional value by 2000 %
- Red/purple berries
- Rhubarb
- Ginger
- Dandelion
- Elderberry

- Chilli Beans, peas, lentils

To sum up this introduction

This introduction to the book has been compiled to give you an over-view of what has been included or excluded in your diet for endometriosis without going into too much scientific detail. The real aim here is to provide you with the recipes to help you feed yourself without the worry of what to cook and what to eat.

As I have said before - these recipes are the absolute bottom line. What this means is that these recipes only include the safest ingredients and recipes for the diet to help minimise the symptoms of endometriosis.

From the feed-back I have received from past readers who have already followed the diet – most of them have said that these recipes are proving to be very popular with other family members, with some dishes becoming family favourites.

So don't worry about feeding the family – just give them some extra protein/red meats if there is a 'man craving his meat' in the house, or you have growing kids. But your health is important here – and if they don't like it – then they know where the kitchen is !!!!

A brief emotional pep talk before we finish ….

What were my personal circumstances and experiences while dealing with endometriosis? – I know some of you will be asking that question. To explain <u>very</u> briefly - my own circumstances were not eased by financial comfort or privilege and being in a secure position to be able to take on this disease. I had many financial issues to deal with, including bailiffs coming to my house as I could not pay my local tax. I had to ration my trips to see my homeopath because of finances. <u>And</u> I had a severe case of endometriosis. Not a great combination of factors to help really. I had to be self-reliant and use will power and determination.

I was, and still am, a realist about this type of healing journey and I am not aiming to mislead anyone. In my own past I had issues to deal with from childhood like abandonment and abuse, and a family not understanding what I was going through with endometriosis and therefore not providing any support. I know that many of you have had to deal with various issues in life, and now being diagnosed with this disease leaves you feeling overwhelmed, helpless, angry, bitter, resentful – just to name a few emotions.

But I have received lots of feedback from other sufferers telling me that they too have been able to reduce their symptoms and regained their health when they chose diet, sometimes combined with other natural treatments.

And lastly ….

We could go into much more detail here about diet and nutrition, and to help I have added links to further reading at the website, which you will find at the back of the book.

If there are any omissions or things you do not understand, you can contact me at the website – how often do you get direct contact with the author! Remember – 'Rome wasn't built in a day' – give this diet a chance to kick in so that you can observe and feel the changes and improvements.

Everyone's healing time will be different. It depends on so many variables:
* The length of time you have been ill
* How deeply the disease has invaded your body
* How toxic your system has become due to hormone drugs, stress overload, pollutants etc.
* The state of your immune system
* Even how much emotional support you get in life can affect healing

Remember what was said earlier, *your immune system is eaves dropping on you* – talk to it kindly and tell yourself you are doing all you can to help fix your body. If you do your bit, your immune system will work with you.

Healing comes from within - and what you put into your body will support your healing

Testimonial:
'Feel free to post my story and e-mail address on your site as you see fit. THANK YOU for your site and THANK YOU for the very informative book and recipes! It's worked miracles for me. THANK YOU!

I've been dealing with endometriosis for over 10 years. I had reduced my sugar and wheat intake for several months when I found your site and recipe book recently, and though I'm normally sceptical about e-books, I downloaded and read it the same night. It's now been eight months since I've eliminated dairy, wheat, sugar, meat, etc. from my diet. It may not work for everyone, but it worked for me. I recently talked to an acquaintance of mine who is also dealing with endometriosis.

She said she would do absolutely anything to reduce her pain. I told her about changing my eating habits, and to my surprise, she said "Oh I could never follow such a strict diet!" I couldn't believe that something as harmless (and beneficial!) as changing your diet wasn't even being considered by someone who had just sworn she'd try anything! Please, if you are looking for an alternative to pain and surgery, PLEASE just TRY the "endometriosis diet" for at least six months. I hate to sound like an infomercial, but I can't stay quiet about my success story when I read about so many people suffering. It might not work, or work as well as it did for me, but what do you have to lose except your pain? Take control.
Erin. USA

Legend/Footnote

I just need to include a few 'translations' here to stop any confusion. There are some differences in the names of certain foods between the US and the UK.

* Spring onions - scallions
* chickpeas - garbanzo
* courgettes - zucchini
* aubergines - eggplants
* coriander – cilantro
* Oestrogen is the spelling in the UK - estrogen in the US

To get an overview of the advice and ingredients used for a diet for endometriosis, I suggest you speed-read through this book. You will then have a better idea of the diet and be able to understand what foods you can and cannot eat.   Also, this process could also give you ideas of how to adjust your own favourite recipes. Sometimes we just need to be shown the way…………..

Eat well and enjoy the benefits.

Yours with healing thoughts

Carolyn Levett

Author/webmistress of www.endo-resolved.com

Recipes

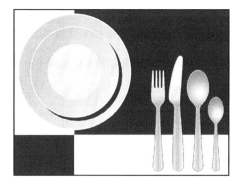

Substitute Ingredients for the endometriosis diet

The diet for Endometriosis advises that you cut out some of the basic ingredients that are normally used in every-day cooking and recipes. This sounds drastic, but fortunately there are alternatives.

Below is a list of alternatives for:

- yoghurt
- milk
- egg - substitute for baking
- sugars
- chocolate
- butter

Nut yoghurts

These will obviously not taste the same as dairy produced yoghurts, but they will have their uses in puddings, and some salad dressings, as an alternative to mayonnaise for that creamy texture required.

Milk substitutes

Milk is a very common ingredient in recipes, but in fact almost any liquid can be used as a substitute. Water, nut and seed milks, fruit juice, or rice milk can be used depending on the recipe. Water can often be used instead of milk. If you want richness, nut milks or rice milk is better. Fruit juice adds sweetness, and rice milk has its own sweetness. Nut and seed milks are very good on cereal, made into healthy milk shakes, or used for cooking in recipes. All have no cholesterol, are low in saturated fat and some are even low in total fat.

You can also make and purchase substitute milk from soy, but I have excluded soy in this book as it is a GM crop, and it is a phytoestrogen plant renowned for the high levels of plant based oestrogen it contains. Please see the Introduction to this book for a further explanation for not using soy in your diet.

Nut and seed milks are also very good in creamy soups, sauces, puddings and ice cream, where the extra richness really makes them special.

By buying in bulk at a warehouse, the cost of making almond milk can be cheaper than cow's milk. Almonds are probably the most nutritious nut. They are higher in calcium than most nuts, and also rich in other nutrients.

Rice and almond milk is available at natural food stores. It is good tasting, rather sweet, and can be used as a substitute in cooking, for drinking, or on cereals.

Fruit juices can be used in your baking to replace milk, especially when extra sweetness is desired. Frozen fruit juice concentrates can be used to replace sugar in recipes if you compensate for the extra liquid.

Egg Substitutes

Eggs are commonly used in baking as a binder to hold dough's together, an important role when the flour you are using contains no gluten. Eggs are helpful in leavening dough, especially useful when baking with whole grain flours.

Commercial egg replacers are available to substitute in your baking. A popular one contains potato starch, tapioca flour and leavening. Others are beginning to appear on the market, but always read the label as some of these will contain egg. These products have been produced as they are meant to lower cholesterol. To use egg replacers, follow the instructions on the packet.

Arrowroot powder is very good for binding dough's when baking. Use about 1 tbs of arrowroot for each 1 cup / 250ml of non-glutinous flour.

Psyllium seed husk powder, the main ingredient in popular bulk laxatives, is usually available in natural food stores. Psyllium provides natural fibre and makes a good binder for breads, cookies, cakes and muffins.

Combine 1 tbs psyllium with 3 tbs water and let the mixture sit for a few minutes before adding to your mixture. Using this small amount in a recipe will not have a strong laxative effect.

If you like bananas, adding half a banana to your cookie, muffin or cake recipe will help to bind the mixture and create a lighter, sweeter and moister result.

If a recipe calls for a single egg (such as a typical batch of cookies or muffins) you can often get away with not using an egg at all, or utilising a single teaspoon of baking powder in its place.

Chocolate Substitute

Carob, sometimes called St. John's Bread, is the fruit of an evergreen tree which can grow to heights of almost 50 feet. Straight from the tree, the fruit looks like a big brown pod. After harvest, it is dried and powdered. Be careful to purchase it raw, because it is generally roasted.

Carob has a flavour similar to chocolate, but without all the negative effects of chocolate. Carob contains Vitamin A and B-complex, minerals, proteins and carbohydrates.

Cacao

Cacao is the raw ingredient for making chocolate and has many health benefits. In the raw state of being uncooked and unprocessed, cacao beans contain a host of health benefits.

Cacao beans are a rich source of various vitamins and minerals. The All-Chocolate website reports 'that raw cacao beans contain healthy amounts of copper and potassium, both of which help to promote heart health, as well as iron, which carries oxygen throughout your body. Cacao beans also contain calcium and magnesium.'

Commercial chocolate contains sugar, milk solids, more milk if its milk chocolate, lecithin, flavourings and preservatives. In other words - lots of bad ingredients that will trigger problems with the symptoms of endometriosis.

Home-made Endo Safe Chocolate
A great recipe I have adapted to be safe for the endometriosis diet

Ingredients:

Raw organic cacao – comes in powder form and can be purchased from many websites, as well as health stores. Some places sell it as little chips of cacao (easily melted)

Coconut oil – most health shops sell this in jars and is also readily available on the internet

Stevia for sweetening

Other flavourings of personal choice – like nuts, ground almonds

Method:

1. Take equal amounts of coconut oil and raw cacao – about 3 or 4 tablespoons of each
2. Melt the coconut oil in a dish like a baine marie (use a porcelain bowl in a pan of hot water) it is not necessary to boil the water because coconut oil melts at 25 degrees
3. Once the coconut oil has melted add the cocoa to the oil and mix well
4. Add a little stevia, about a quarter teaspoon – add this to taste because the strength of stevia can differ
5. To provide the equivalent solidity that is found with commercial chocolate, add some 'fibre'/ bulking agent, and one good method is to add grated coconut, this gives it a bit more bite. You will need about one large tablespoon. You can use dried grated coconut or fresh coconut.

You can add all sorts of nice things - small pieces of chopped dates, chopped up nuts. This is the stage you can experiment with.

When you're done, pour your mixture into small dishes or ice cube trays. Put the mixture in the refrigerator. When the coconut oil is completely set it is ready to eat. The chocolate will melt when out of the refrigerator, because coconut oil has a low melting point, so keep it in the fridge.

This recipe can also be used to make chocolate sauce in the runny state – yummy! Add it to puddings or poured over endo safe cake recipes – how naughty is that!

Recipes and Tips for Alternative Ingredients

Some of these ingredients can now be purchased from your health store. These recipes are included to provide you with options and in some instances can save you money.

Almond Yoghurt

Ingredients:

2 cups / 500ml sprouted almonds, blanched

12 oz / 350ml filtered water

Method:

1. Put the sprouted almonds into a blender with the water and blend to a fine cream.
2. Pour the cream into a muslin bag and squeeze out all the liquid. You should have approx. 10 oz / 300ml Put this liquid into a wide- mouth glass jar, cover with muslin or cheesecloth and let it sit at room temperature for 8 hours. The yoghurt will separate from the whey, which stays on the bottom of the jar.
3. When done, put the jar into the refrigerator and let it solidify more. To serve, scoop out the yoghurt from the top CAREFULLY, so as not to mix the yoghurt with the whey.

Makes approximately 6 oz / 175g of yoghurt. Keeps for up to 5 days in the refrigerator.

When storing all nut and seed yoghurts, keep them in the same glass jar that you made them in, but when screwing on the top, leave it loose. In other words; do not screw the top on tight. This lets in a little air circulation and doesn't build up any pressure in the jar and the yoghurt lasts longer.

Pine Nut Yoghurt

Ingredients:

2 cups / 500ml pine nuts

8 oz / 220ml filtered water

Additional filtered water for soaking

Method:

1. Soak the pine nuts in filtered water for 8 hours. Rinse, drain and sprout for 8 hours.

2. Rinse again. Put the nuts into a blender with 7-8 oz / 200 – 220ml filtered water and blend to a fine cream.

3. Pour the cream into a muslin bag and squeeze out all the liquid. There should be approx. 12 oz / 350ml of liquid. Put the liquid into a wide-mouth glass jar, cover with cheesecloth or muslin cloth, and let sit at room temperature for 8 hours (5-7 hours in hot weather). You will see the whey separate from the cream, which rises to the top.

4. Then it is done, put into the refrigerator for about 3 hours, so the cream solidifies more. To serve, scoop out the yoghurt carefully as needed from the top, leaving the whey on the bottom of the jar.

Yield: approx. 1 cup / 250ml of a very rich and tasty yoghurt. Keeps for up to 5 days in the refrigerator.

Note about alternative milks: You can now buy a variety of dairy free milks at many health stores including almond milk, thin coconut milk, rice milk. So you do have options

Basic Nut Milk Recipe

Ingredients:

½ cup / 150ml nuts

2 cups / 500ml water

Method:

Put nuts in blender container. Process until nuts are finely ground. Add ½ cup / 150ml water and blend on low speed for a few seconds, then turn the blender up high. Blend for a couple of minutes.

Gradually add another 1½ cups / 400ml of water to the mix and blend well. Put milk in a covered jar and store in refrigerator. It will keep 4 to 5 days.

Variations: You can use raw walnuts, cashews, pecans, brazil nuts, almonds, sunflower seeds, pumpkins seeds, sesame seeds, and other nuts and seeds to make milk using the same technique. Use the same proportions of nut to water, ½ cup / 65g nuts to 2 cups / 500ml of water. If the milk seems grainy, strain through cheesecloth. Let it stand for a few minutes draining through cloth, then squeeze out milk from pulp.

Almond Milk - using sprouted almonds

Makes almost a quart / 2 pints

Ingredients:

1 cup / 130g sprouted almonds, blanched

3 ½ cups / 900ml filtered water

Method:

1. Process almonds in the blender with ½ to 1 cups / 150ml to 250ml of water until well blended, then add balance of water and blend again.

2. Pour into a cotton or muslin bag or cloth and squeeze out all the milk. This is simple, plain almond milk. This milk can be enjoyed as is or flavoured in various ways.

3. Keeps for up to 5 days in the refrigerator. After storage, the milk separates - so shake well before using. Save the leftover almond pulp to make cookies.

Rice Milk

Ingredients:

1 cup / 130g hot, fresh cooked rice (white or brown)

4 cups / 1000ml hot water

Pinch of salt (optional)

Sweetener to taste (if desired)

Vanilla to taste (if desired)

Method:

Put in blender and process until creamy. Strain it through a cheesecloth or other cloth with tiny holes. Discard solids (you may want to use these as a thickener in a soup or stew). Store rice milk in jar in refrigerator it will keep 3-4 days. Make sure to shake it before using!

Oat Milk - with Added Flavour

Ingredients:

4 cups / 1000ml (cold) water

1 ripe banana

2 cups / 260g cooked oatmeal

1 tsp. vanilla

Pinch of salt (opt.)

1 tsp vanilla (opt.)

Sweetener to taste (if desired)

Method:

Place all ingredients in blender and process until smooth

Additional Egg Replacements

In most baking, eggs provide a binding and a rising agent - so whatever you use to replace them has to provide some liquid and something to create the rising effect. Each of the recipes below is the equivalent of one egg (except the flax seed recipe).

Applesauce: Add about ¼ / 70ml cup with a 1/2 tsp of baking powder.

Banana: Use ½ banana, mashed with ½ teaspoon of baking soda. This is good for recipes that would benefit with a banana taste.

Baking powder: Add an extra ½ teaspoon baking powder and about 2-4 tablespoons extra liquid to replace one egg in a recipe.

Flax seed: This flax seed mixture can be used in place of 2 eggs: Grind 3 tablespoons flax seed to a very fine powder in a blender. Add ½ / 150ml cup water and blend until the mixture becomes thick, resembling raw egg whites. Fold it into cake batter at the end of mixing for light vegan cakes, but only use in recipes that call for 2 or 3 eggs at the most.

Butter/Margarine Alternatives

In sauces or baking, generally it is very easy to use vegetable oils instead of solid fats. For baking, your best bet is to use sunflower oil or other organic oils from nuts and seeds. When making sauces that call for butter or margarine, olive oil always works just fine (and adds a nicer flavour).

If you are looking to replace margarine on vegetables - try flax seed oil - you can't cook with this oil, but it does make a good salad dressing and contains many essential nutrients for your body.

Nut Butter

Nut butters are very easily made in the food processor. Once made they can be thinned with a little oil and flavoured with herbs, spices and vegetables for savoury applications. They can also be mixed with fruit purees, chopped dates or bananas to make cake fillings, sweet spreads or fruit stuffing.

Suitable nuts are hazelnuts, walnuts and peanuts. Cashew nuts can also be used but they tend to remain much dryer without the addition of extra oil.

Ingredients:

1 ½ cups / 250g nuts

A little nut oil

Method:
Remove the skins from the nuts if necessary and blend in a food processor for a few minutes until the ground nuts start to exude their oils and stick together. Add a little more oil at this stage as necessary.

Note: Some health shops now sell various nut butters

Varieties of Alternative Sweeteners

On a diet for Endometriosis, one of the ingredients to cut down to a minimum is sugar. The regime for a diet to combat Candida is to eliminate sugar intake.

There is too much sugar in the average Western diet and it can be found in surprising places in convenience foods. Table sugar is usually made from beets, corn, or cane (a relative of wheat), or a blend of all three.

Following a healthy diet to eliminate sugar becomes difficult to if you want to include sweets/puddings, baking, and cakes in your diet, or you prefer sweetener in your drinks.

There are fortunately other alternatives that do not have the same ill health effects as sugar. If you shop at natural food stores, you will find a wide variety of natural sweeteners. Under no circumstances should you replace sugar with artificial sweeteners.

When baking cookies, muffins, and cakes, try adding fruit juice, dates, bananas, or fruit puree to replace the sweetness required in your recipe.

Aspartame - (NutriSweet) – Don't use this one. I have included this information as a warning. Asparame forms methanol and formaldehyde in the body and can cause numerous side effects. Saccharin sweeteners are weak carcinogens. Fructose, used comprehensively in convenience foods, is not made from fruit, as you might suppose, but it is a highly refined product made from table sugar and may contain corn.

Amasake - Amasake is a traditional Japanese product made by fermenting sweet brown rice into a thick liquid. It is a creamy, quickly digested beverage used by athletes after a workout or as a sweetener in cooking or baking

Brown rice syrup - Brown rice syrup is a naturally processed sweetener, made from sprouted brown rice. It is thick and mild-flavoured.

Date sugar - can be used on those occasions when you need a dry sugar. It is made from ground dates and is usually available from natural food stores. Try it in your crumble mix for fruit crumbles.

Fruit juice concentrates - Fruit juice concentrates are made by cooking down various fruits, grape, and pear juices to produce a sweeter, more concentrated product. The product is then frozen to increase shelf life.

Honey - is often suggested in many recipes, but honey is another food that should not be used by women with endometriosis unless they can be sure that the honey they purchase is certified organic honey.

You need to be aware of not buying contaminated imported honey, which can be diluted or contaminated with antibiotics and other chemicals. Also it has been found that some honey is obtained from bees that are using pollen from GM crops to produce honey. And finally, honey can be filtered so much during processing that there is no beneficial pollen left in the honey, thus leaving it with no nutritional value.

Maple syrup - and rice syrup can be used the same way as you would use honey in your diet. Maple syrup contains fewer calories and a higher concentration of minerals than honey. It is available throughout the year in your local supermarket. Get the best quality you can.

Stevia - is another great sugar alternative and is now being sold in many supermarkets and health shops. It is a plant which is native to Paraguay. Stevia is 30 times sweeter than sugar. Studies have found the leaf to contain proteins, fibre, carbohydrates, iron, phosphorus, calcium, potassium, sodium, magnesium, zinc, rutin (a flavonoid), true vitamin A, Vitamin C and an oil which contains 53 other constituents. Do not purchase Stevia from the supermarket as this is usually a poor quality product, and it is better to purchase from your local health store.

Buying and Storing Tips

Liquid alternative sweeteners (amasake, barley malt, brown rice syrup, and maple syrup) can be stored at room temperature in the original packaging until opened, but should be refrigerated after opening. Dry, powdered alternative sweeteners should be stored in a dry place at room temperature. Fruit juice concentrates should remain frozen until ready to use.

Preparation, uses, and tips

Alternative sweeteners are used to sweeten hot and cold beverages, and are used in place of refined sweeteners in cooking and baking. Most dry, powdered alternative sweeteners are easily substituted for white sugar (1 part for 1 part) in recipes.

When using a liquid sweetener in place of sugar, reduce the liquid content in the recipe by ¼ cup / 65ml. If the recipe calls for no liquid, add 3 to 5 tbsp (22.5 to 37.5g) of flour for each ¾ cup (200ml) of liquid sweetener.

Baking Powder

Commercial baking powders usually contain corn-starch and other unwanted ingredients to prevent caking. It is easy and economical to make your own baking powder. The basic ingredients are cream of tartar and baking soda. Arrowroot powder is added to help keep it free-flowing. If the mixture cakes, mash it with your fingers.

To make your own baking powder, mix together 2 parts cream of tartar, 1 part baking soda, and 2 parts arrowroot powder. Store in an airtight container, and substitute any recipe calling for baking powder.

Soy Sauce

Soy sauce is often used as a salt substitute or flavouring for Chinese food. Soy is usually a GM crop and is well known for the high levels of phytoestrogens, which women with Endometriosis need to consume in a balanced manner (please see Introduction about balancing your phytoestrogen intake)

All soy contains considerable amounts of sodium. Use wheat-free, preservative free tamari sauce instead of soy sauce. Tamari is very similar to soy sauce, but is a higher quality product, which is why I have included it in this book as an ingredient to use in your savoury cooking.

Please see the Introduction for more information about Soy.

Gelatine

Gelatine is made from animal products - usually from the bones and hoofs of animals. It is used as a setting agent in sweets like jellies.

Agar-agar, made from seaweed is a good substitute. It is high in fibre and contains many vitamins and minerals.

One tablespoon of granulated agar-agar or 2 tablespoons of flaked agar-agar will gel about 2 cups / 500ml of liquid. Either will substitute for 1 tablespoons of gelatine.

Breakfast Ideas

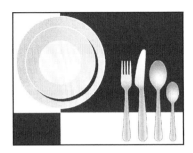

- Gluten or wheat free cereal with non-dairy milk, such as rice milk or coconut milk – most health food stores are now selling a great variety of gluten or wheat free breakfast cereals.
- Porridge made from oats using non-dairy milk like coconut milk
- Fruit smoothies
- Plain and simple - cut up fruit, you can add some 'live' yoghurt for extra health benefits and nuts
- Rice pudding- you can make a simple version by heating up some pre-cooked brown rice with either rice milk or coconut milk and add some cinnamon if you like
- Lightly fried mushrooms and tomatoes served on wheat free toast
- Home-made hash browns, or bubble and squeak
- *Gluten free* pancakes with some yoghurt and maple syrup – make the pancakes with egg re-placer – you can use eggs as long as they are organic.

Hot Drinks

Some drinks are measured in 'parts' (ie – one teaspoon/part is a good strength) depending how strong you want to make these warming drinks. Also the amount of water used will affect strength, but you will only want to make sufficient herb teas for one or two drinks each time.

Simple Chai

Ingredients:

1½ cups/ 400ml water

½ inch cinnamon stick

4 cardamom pods

4 cloves

Method:

Put the water in a pan. Add the ingredients and bring to a boil. Cover, turn heat to low and simmer for 10 minutes. Strain the tea into cup and serve immediately.

Hot Chocolate

Ingredients:

¾ cup / 200ml pure coconut milk

¼ cup / 70ml water (If you use lite coconut milk DO NOT ADD WATER.)

½ tbs carob powder

Maple syrup to taste

Method:

Combine coconut milk, water and carob powder. Blend with a wire whisk, heat on stove top. Add maple syrup to taste

"Coffee Substitute"

Ingredients:

2 cups/ 500ml water

1 tbs roasted chicory root

1 tbs dried dandelion root (not roasted)

½ tsp cardamom seed (should be out of the husk, but not ground)

Method:

Put water in a pan. Add roasted chicory root, dandelion root, and cardamom seed. Simmer gently 10 minutes. Strain and enjoy. I have found this is pretty pleasant to drink. No it doesn't taste exactly like coffee but it is dark and tasty and pretty good for you.

Warming Winter Spice Tea

Ingredients:

½ part cinnamon bark or powdered cinnamon

½ part dried ginger-root

½ part (hulled) cardamom seeds

½ part star anise

Maple syrup to taste

Method:

Slowly heat 4 cups / 1000ml of water in a pot. Put the ingredients, except maple syrup, into a mortar and with a pestle crush the herbs slightly. Or put them in a blender and turn it on briefly, just enough to release some of the aromas. Add the herbs to the water and let it stand to infuse for a few minutes. Strain and add maple syrup to taste if required.

Cold Weather Tea

Infuse together:

1 part roasted dandelion root

1 part ginger-root 1 part cinnamon bark

½ part liquorice root

½ part prickly ash bark

Warm yourself with the circulation-supporting herbs in this blend.

Vitamin C-Rich Tea

Infuse together:

1 part dandelion leaf

1 part rose hip

1 part hibiscus flower

1 part raspberry leaf

These vitamin C-rich herbs are also high in flavonoids, which help improve the body's assimilation of that nutrient.

Pain Relief Tea

Ingredients:

2 cups / 500ml of water

1 tsp grated fresh ginger root
1 tsp raspberry leaves
1 tsp Maple syrup if desired
Bring water to a boil. Place herbs in water and stir. Turn heat to
low and simmer for 15 minutes.

Method:

Ginger has both pain relieving and anti-nausea properties. Raspberry leaves have uterine relaxant properties and help relieve diarrhoea. This is a helpful combination for relief of endometriosis symptoms

Post-surgery/Recovery Tea

Infuse together:

1 part dandelion leaf

1 part nettle leaf

1 part dandelion root

½ part liquorice root

1 part Siberian ginseng root

This is an excellent blend for cleansing drug residue out of the body and building strength and energy.

Spiced Green Tea

Add to your cup of green tea:

4 to 8 cloves

A dash of cinnamon

Maple Syrup to taste

Dried orange peel pieces (optional)

Cold Drinks

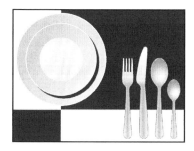

Apple Lemonade

Makes about 2 servings

Ingredients:

2 cups / 500ml un-sweetened apple juice

4 tablespoons pure lemon juice

Method:

Combine juices. Chill. Serve over ice.

Cantaloupe Smoothie

Take half a cantaloupe, clean and peel it, and slice it up into chunks. Then put it in a blender, with 4-6 ice cubes and enough water to cover the cantaloupe. (If you have a small blender, you can use smaller amounts of everything.) Then blend it on HIGH for about a minute. When it's whipped up, it has a sweet, creamy consistency, which is perfect for anybody who craves drinking milk.

Coconut Milk

In a blender or food processor, combine ½ cup / 150ml each grated un-sweetened coconut and boiling water. Blend until coconut is finely ground. Strain through a fine sieve or a piece of clean muslin, squeezing to extract all the liquid. Discard coconut. Makes about ½ cup / 150ml.

Healing Smoothie

This is a great drink for anyone, especially those with ulcers. This drink has soothing qualities which protect and heal the stomach lining.

Ingredients:

1 firm kiwi fruit, peeled

¼ cantaloupe, with skin

1 ripe banana

Method:

Process kiwi fruit and cantaloupe through a juice extractor.

Place juice and banana in a blender or food processor and blend until smooth.

Orange and Papaya Shake

This juicing recipe will act as an aid for indigestion.

Ingredients:

1 orange, peeled (leave white pithy part on)

½ papaya peeled

1 banana

Orange twist for garnish

Method:

Juice orange with papaya. Place juice and banana into a blender or food processor, and blend until smooth. Garnish with the orange twist.

Strawberry - Banana Smoothie

Ingredients:

3 tbs blanched almonds
1 cup / 250ml water or apple juice
2 dates, pitted
2/3rds cup strawberries, fresh or frozen
1 banana, peeled, and broken into 2-inch pieces

Method:

In a blender, place the almonds, and process for 30 seconds to finely chop. Scrape down the sides of the blender container, add the water and dates, and process for 1 minute. Add the remaining ingredients and process an additional 1-2 minutes or until smooth and creamy. Serve immediately

Variation: substitute other fruit or berries in the recipe, as desired.

Iced Lemon Mint Green Tea

Get the benefits of Green Tea in this refreshing and cooling drink. Green Tea made the usual way as a hot drink does not suit everyone's taste so this chilled version is a good alternative.

Ingredients:

5 cups / 1250ml water, divided
4 tsp green tea leaf
1 cup / 250ml lemon juice
1/3rd cup / 80ml brown rice syrup
¼ cup / 70ml freshly chopped mint
Garnishes: ice cubes, lemon slices, and sprigs of mint

Method:

In a small saucepan, bring 3 cups water and tea to a boil, remove the saucepan from the heat, and set aside for 5 minutes to allow the tea to steep. Strain the tea, and allow the tea to cool completely.

In a pitcher/jug, combine the brewed tea and the remaining 2 cups water / 500ml, along with the remaining ingredients, except for the garnishes, and stir well to combine. Place the pitcher in the refrigerator and allow the mixture to chill for 30 minutes or more to allow the flavours to blend. Serve in ice-filled glasses and garnish each with a lemon slice and sprig of mint.

Home-Made Strawberry Lemonade

Ingredients:

8 cups / 2000ml water

1 cup / 130g fresh-cut strawberries

1 cup / 130g frozen strawberries

Maple syrup to taste

1 cup / 250ml lemon juice

2 lemons sliced

Method:

1. In a large container, combine 4 cups / 1000ml of water and the fresh and frozen strawberries.

Soak for 3-4 hours.

2. In another container, combine the lemon juice, sliced lemons and water. Chill for 3-4 hours to let the lemon juice soak through. Mix the 2 containers together, and add maple syrup to your taste. Serve chilled over ice.

Pink Drink

Ingredients:

1 quart / 1150ml spearmint or other tea

½ quart / 600ml fresh apple cider

½ quart / 600ml grape juice

Juice of 2 lemons

Method:

Maple syrup to taste

Put in a large punch bowl with thin slices of lemon floating. Plenty for a large group.

Frosty Punch

Ingredients:

1 quart / 1150ml pineapple juice, un-sweetened

1 cup / 130g fresh or frozen cranberries

2 sprigs of mint

Method:

Blend all ingredients together until smooth

Strawberry Fruit Drink

Ingredients:

2 cups / 500ml pineapple juice

2 cups / 250g fresh strawberries

1 banana, or 1 cup / 130g diced mango, or 1 cup / 130g diced peaches

Method:

Blend together until smooth.

Fruity Summer Cooler

Ingredients:

6-8 ice cubes

½ cup / 65g cubed cantaloupe

½ cup / 65g pineapple chunks

½ cup / 65g cranberry juice

1/3rd cup / 45g sliced banana

¼ cup / 70ml pineapple juice

Maple syrup to taste

¾ tsp lemon juice

Method:

Blend all ingredients until smooth.

Basic Fruit Smoothie

Ingredients:

1 cup / 250ml apple juice, unsweetened

1 peeled frozen banana

½ cup / 70g of frozen favourite fruit (strawberries, melons, blueberries, peaches) Add more if you want it thicker

Method:

Put apple juice into blender, add banana cut into chunks. Blend until creamy. Add second fruit of choice, and blend again.

Another Smoothie

Ingredients:

1 cup / 250ml pineapple juice

1 peeled frozen banana

½ cup / 70g frozen strawberries

2 pitted dates

Method:

Blend all ingredients until smooth

Note: *You can adjust the amounts of juice and fruit to make them thicker or thinner as desired*

Soups

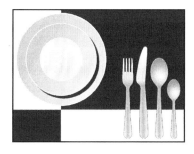

Soups are brilliant. In most recipes, once you have done all the chopping, you simple chuck all the ingredients into one pan and leave it to simmer until cooked. If you add less liquid, then soups can provide a meal by themselves, just add some fresh home-baked bread (non-wheat based of course) and you have a complete meal.

Pick recipes where the vegetables are in season to help keep cost down. Most soup recipes will freeze well, and to save on time, effort, and power consumption simple increase the amount of ingredients to cook up a big pot full of soup, which you can eat some immediately and freeze the rest.

Cream of Cauliflower Soup

Serves 4-6

Ingredients:

A large head of cauliflower

2-3 stalks celery

1 carrot

2 cloves garlic

1-2 onions

1-2 tsp ground cumin

½ tsp pepper a few sprigs of parsley

¼ tsp sage (or your favourite blend of herbs; spices)

Method:

1. Chop head of cauliflower (save a handful of tiny flowerets for a raw garnish) and put in a saucepan.
2. Chop and add stalks celery, carrot, garlic and onions and add spices.
3. Barely cover with water, bring to boil and simmer until veggies are tender.
4. Let cool a little then blend with a food blender and adjust seasonings to taste.
5. Add a little hot water if the soup is too thick. Serve garnished with raw flowerets.

You can use the same basic recipe for Cream of Broccoli, Cream of Courgette or Cream of Asparagus Soup. You won't miss the fact that there is no actual cream in the soup, given the thick consistency and rich flavour of the main veggie. You can also add a little milk substitute in place of extra water to make the soup more even more creamy.

Cream of Coconut and Mango Soup

Serves 6 – plenty of servings for parties/catering or freezing

This is a cold soup with a blend of wonderful fruity flavours. You do not have to use all the flavourings in this recipe if you find if difficult to purchase them. You can omit the lemon-grass and use a squeeze of lemon juice instead. Use vanilla essence instead of using fresh vanilla for a cheaper option.

Ingredients:

2-3 tablespoons arrowroot

1/8th cup / 35ml water

4 cups / 1000ml fresh coconut milk

1/8th cup / 35ml organic honey or sweetener of choice

2 cardamom pods

1 stalk lemon grass, bruised

3 quarter-size pieces ginger-root, bruised

1 vanilla bean, split

½ cup / 150ml cream of coconut

3 cups / 450g mango (3 mangos)

½ -inch diced ginger

2 tbs fresh-squeezed orange juice

2 tbs fresh-squeezed lime juice

1 tbs rice syrup

Garnish: fresh mint sprigs

Method:

1. In a saucepan set over moderate heat, combine coconut milk, rice syrup, cardamom pods, lemon grass, ginger and vanilla. Bring to a simmer for 10 minutes then let cool. Chill, covered, overnight.
2. In a bowl, combine the arrowroot with the water. Strain the chilled coconut mixture.
3. In a saucepan set over moderate heat, combine the arrowroot with the coconut milk mixture, bring to a simmer and cook over low heat, stirring frequently, for 10 minutes, or until thicken then leave to cool.
4. In a separate bowl, combine mango with orange juice, lime juice and rice syrup. Then mix into the coconut cream when it is cooled. Serve garnished with mint leaves

Cream of Mushroom Soup

Serves 2 - 3

Ingredients:

1 avocado

1 tomato

1 cup / 250ml hot water

1 red (bell) sweet pepper (diced)

1 cup / 130g mushrooms (sliced)

1 little onion (diced)

1 clove of garlic

Juice of half grapefruit,

Chopped basil

Sea salt to taste

Method:

In a food blender, blend together avocado, grapefruit juice, garlic and hot water. Then add sliced mushrooms, sweet pepper, tomato, onion, salt and basil. You may choose any of your favourite vegetables as an addition to this soup.

It can be served as a 'raw' cold soup straight from the blender, which is packed full of goodness. If you prefer you can heat the mixture for a warm soup, but it is nicer eaten cold.

Cream of Tomato Soup

Serves 4

Ingredients:

2 large potatoes, scrubbed and chopped

1 can tomatoes or 1 cup chopped tomatoes

2 tbs tomato pure

½ tsp dried basil

1 tsp mixed herbs dried

1 tsp paprika

Sea salt to taste

1 cup / 250ml rice milk

Juice of 1 lemon

Method:

1. Place all the ingredients except lemon juice into a large saucepan. Bring to the boil, cover and simmer until potatoes are soft.
2. Blend in food processor or blender until smooth, adding lemon juice to taste.

Red Gazpacho Soup

Serves 6 – 8 – keeps well in the refrigerator for a few days

This is a classic cold soup recipe that is blended together in a food blender. It is best prepared the day before eating to allow all the flavours to blend together.

Ingredients:

1 bell pepper, chopped

3 med. tomatoes, peeled and chopped

1 cucumber, peeled and chopped

1 small onion, chopped

2 tbs olive oil

Dash pepper

Dash paprika

Shake of Tabasco

2 ½ cups / 650ml tomato juice

1 tsp. chives

2 tsp. parsley

½ clove garlic, minced

4 ½ tsp. lemon juice

Method:

Mix all ingredients together in a blender, and refrigerate at least 12 hours.

Courgette Soup

Serves 3 - 4

Ingredients:

1 large onion, chopped

2 tbs olive oil

2 cups / 500ml vegetable stock

8 cups / 1200g diced courgette

 - about 3 to 4 medium courgettes

2 cloves garlic, chopped

1/8th tsp celery salt

Dash of pepper

¼ cup / 30g parsley leaves

Method:

1. In a pan, sauté onion in oil until tender.

2. Add remaining ingredients except parsley. Cook over medium heat about 5 minutes or until courgettes are tender.

3. Carefully pour into blender or food processor, and add parsley and blend until smooth. May be thinned with additional stock. Serve hot or cold.

Butterbean and herb cream soup

Serves 6

Ingredients:

6 cups / 1500ml water or vegetable stock
2 ½ cups / 450g butter beans, sorted, and rinsed
1 bay leaf
¼ cup / 30g freshly chopped basil
¼ cup / 30g freshly chopped Italian parsley
2 tbs. freshly chopped dill
½ tsp salt
¼ tsp freshly ground black pepper

Method:

1. In a large pot, combine the water, butter beans, and bay leaf, and bring to a boil. Reduce the heat to low, cover, and simmer the beans until tender about 1 - 1 ½ hours.

2. Remove the pot of beans from the heat and remove and discard the bay leaf. Using a blender or food processor, process the beans and their cooking liquid to form a smooth puree. Add the remaining ingredients and process a few times to combine. Taste and adjust the seasonings, if needed.

You may need to return soup to pan to bring back to required heat.

Curried Apple Soup

Serves 6 - 8 Can be served hot or cold

Ingredients:

1 cup / 130g spring onions, finely diced
2 tbs safflower oil
1 tbs. curry powder
2 tsp ginger, minced
¼ cup / 70ml sherry (optional)

3 lbs / 1300g cooking apples of choice -
peeled, cored, and diced
4 cups / 1000ml vegetable stock
1 cup / 250ml apple juice
1 cup / 250ml non-dairy milk
1-2 tbs lemon juice
salt and pepper, to taste

Method:

1. In a large pot, sauté the spring onions in oil for 5 minutes or until soft. Add the curry powder and ginger, and cook an additional minute. Add the sherry, and stir well.

2. Add the diced apples, vegetable stock, and apple juice, and bring the mixture to a boil. Cover, reduce the heat to low, and simmer for 15 - 20 minutes or until the apples are tender.

3. Remove from the heat and allow to cool for 10 minutes. In a food processor or blender, in batches, puree the soup until smooth, and return the soup to the pot. Whisk in the milk, a little of the lemon juice, and season to taste with salt and pepper.

If desired, add additional curry powder, apple juice, or lemon juice to the soup to adjust the sweetness or spicy flavour of the soup to your own personal taste. Serve hot or cold.

Winter Squash Bisque

Serves 6 – 8 – Suitable for catering or freezing

Ingredients:

1½ cups / 200g onion, diced
1 cup / 60g (about ¾ med) spring onions, sliced
3 tbs olive oil
3 lbs. butternut (or other winter squash), peeled - de-seeded, and cut into 1-inch cubes
1 tbs ginger, minced
7 cups / 1750ml vegetable stock
½ cup / 150ml orange juice
1 tbs. orange zest
½ tsp cinnamon
½ tsp salt

¼ tsp nutmeg
1 bay leaf
1 cup / 250ml rice milk, or other non-dairy milk
Garnishes: toasted pumpkin seeds or toasted almonds, or freshly snipped chives

Method:

1. In a large pot, sauté the onion and spring onion in olive oil for 5 minutes to soften. Add the butternut squash and ginger, and cook an additional 5 minutes. Add the vegetable stock, orange juice, orange zest, cinnamon, salt, nutmeg, and bay leaf, and bring to a boil. Cover, reduce heat to low, and simmer for 25 minutes or until the squash is tender.

2. Remove the pot from the heat, remove the bay leaves, and discard them. Using a blender or food processor, puree the soup in batches. Stir in the milk and reheat the soup until just heated through, if necessary. Do not boil the soup or the milk will curdle. Garnish individual servings with a few toasted pumpkin seeds or toasted almonds, or a few snipped chives for colour.

Light Vegetable Soup

Serves 2 - 3

 Ingredients:

2/3rds tbs oil
¼ cup / 30g (about ½ onion) diced onion

1 cup / 130g thinly sliced carrots

1 cup / 130g thinly sliced courgette

2 tsp chopped fresh parsley

¼ tsp thyme

1/8th tsp pepper

3 cups / 750ml veg stock

Method:

1. In a medium saucepan, cook onion in oil until translucent; add all other ingredients except stock. Cover and cook over low heat, stirring occasionally, until vegetables are tender, about 10 - 15 minutes. Add stock and bring to boil

2. Remove about a ¼ of the soup from pan and reserve; pour remaining soup into blender and process at low speed until smooth. Combine pureed and reserved mixtures in saucepan and cook, stirring constantly until hot.

Pesto Soup

Serves 4

This is another cold soup that involves no cooking. All the ingredients are blended together in a food processor or blender

Ingredients:

½ cup / 50g pine nuts soaked overnight, rinsed

10-12 medium size ripe and soft juicy tomatoes, quartered

Large bunch of basil leaves, washed and striped

1 inch ginger, partly chopped up

1 avocado, skinned a stone removed - roughly chopped

Juice of 2 lemons

Bunch of chives - roughly chopped

Method:

Mix and liquefy all ingredients in a blender
If this is too much for your blender, split it up into 2 batches

Serve with a sprig of Basil or Parsley

Indian Bean Soup

Serves 4-6

A thick and hearty soup, nourishing and substantial enough to serve as a main meal with chunks of wheat-free bread. Black-eye beans are used here, but red kidney beans may be added to the mixture if preferred. This is an ideal recipe to put some aside for freezing.

Ingredients:

4 tbs oil

2 onions, chopped

1½ cups / 250g potato, cut into chunks

1½ cups / 250g parsnip, cut into chunks

1½ cups / 250g turnip or swede, cut into chunks

2 celery sticks, trimmed and sliced

2 courgettes, trimmed and sliced

1 green (bell) pepper, cut into ½ inch pieces

2 garlic cloves, crushed

2 tsp ground coriander

1 tbs paprika

1 tbs mild curry paste

2 pints / 1130ml vegetable stock

15oz / 420g can black-eye beans,

(drained and rinsed)

Sea salt

Method:

1. Heat the oil in a saucepan, add all the prepared vegetables except the courgettes, and cook over a moderate heat for 5 mins, stirring frequently. Add the garlic, coriander, paprika and curry paste and cook for 1 minute, stirring.

2. Stir in the stock and seasoning with salt to taste. Bring to the boil, cover and simmer gently for 20 mins, stirring occasionally.

3. Stir in the black-eye beans and sliced courgettes, cover and continue cooking for a further 12 mins or until all the vegetables are tender.

4. Puree ½ pint / 280ml of the soup mixture in a food processor or blender. Return the pureed mixture to the soup in the saucepan and reheat until piping hot. Sprinkle with chopped coriander.

The flavour of the soup improves if it is made the day before eating, as this allows time for all the flavours to blend and develop

Spicy Lentil Soup

4 servings - You can never go wrong with a good spicy lentil soup – it's almost a meal in itself

Ingredients:

2 tbs oil

1 onion, chopped

2 celery sticks, chopped

2 carrots, chopped

Garlic

½ cup / 110g red lentils, rinsed

1 pint / 560ml vegetable stock

Salt and pepper

Curry powder

Method:

1. In a pan, cook onion, carrot, and celery with a little oil till soft. Add remaining ingredients, bring to the boil and simmer for 45 minutes, stirring occasionally. There is no need to blend this soup as the lentils will break down, but if you want a smooth soup you can blend it to break down the veggies.

2. Check seasoning. Serve with a swirl of nut yoghurt and chopped coriander leaves

Parsnip and Brown Rice Soup

Serves 4 - 6

Ingredients:

3 medium parsnips, scrubbed and chopped small

1 medium onion, chopped

2 tbs olive oil

1 tsp cumin seeds

4 cups / 1000ml water

½ cup / 150ml tamari

2 cups cooked brown rice - i.e. 1 cup / 450g raw

Method:

1. Place all ingredients, except rice, in a heavy based pan, bring to boil, then reduce heat and simmer for about 35 minutes, until the parsnips are very tender.

2. Stir the cooked rice into the rest of the ingredients and heat. Serve immediately.

Lentil Squash Soup

Serves: 6-8 - *Bulk cooking recipe - ideal for freezing*

Ingredients:

3 cups / 600g red lentils

1-2 kg squash, orange, big variety

1 onion - chopped

1 red pepper - chopped

Vegetable stock

2 tsp olive oil

Sea salt to taste

Cayenne pepper to taste

1 lemon - juiced for seasoning

3 cloves garlic, finely chopped

Method:

1. Rinse lentils well, cover with water, season and simmer about 20 minutes or until lentils are quite soft.

2. In the meantime chop onion and red pepper. Fry in small amount of olive oil.

3. Peel squash and cut into cubes of about 4cm or so. Put into the pot with the onion and red pepper. Usually the squash has enough water in it. Close lid well and wait for a while before you stir for the first time. If you don't smell anything burning, everything is fine, otherwise add some water. After about an hour, the squash should be soft.

4. Mix with lentils and blend everything. If the result is too thick, add water.

5. Season with garlic, lemon juice, cayenne pepper, salt to taste.

Tomato, Carrot and Lentil Soup

Serves 4 – 6

Ingredients:

2 large onions, chopped

2 cups / 400g fresh tomatoes

4 medium carrots, grated

5 cups / 1250ml vegetable stock

4 tsp tomato puree

¾ cup / 150g split red lentils

1 bay leaf

1 tsp turmeric

1 heaped tsp cumin

Freshly ground black pepper to taste

Method:

1. Soften the onion, tomatoes and carrots in the stock and tomato puree for 5 minutes over a gentle heat.
2. Add lentils, spices and seasoning. Cover and bring to the boil. Turn down heat and simmer for 40 minutes
3. Serve chunky or put through a food processor or blender to make a smooth soup.
4. Add a couple of handfuls of brown rice to make a quick and easy meal.

Curried Parsnip and Lentil Soup

Serves 4 - 6

Ingredients:

2 tbs olive oil

1 large onion, chopped

2 large parsnips, peeled and chopped

1¾ pint / 1000ml vegetable stock

1 - 2 tsp curry powder

Sea salt and freshly ground black pepper to taste

1 cups / 120g red lentils

Paprika to garnish

Method:

1. Heat the oil in a heavy pan, and cook the chopped onion until soft. Add the parsnips, stock, curry powder, seasoning, and lentils. Cover the pan and simmer on a low heat until the parsnips and lentils are cooked (about 40 minutes).
2. Remove from the heat, and processes in a blender until smooth.
3. Return to the pan, reheat and serve immediately.

Nutmeg Carrot Soup

Serves 4

Ingredients:

1 tbs olive oil

3 to 4 med carrots

1 large potato

1 medium onion

2½ cups / 650ml vegetable stock

¼ cup / 30g whole-grain rice

Freshly ground nutmeg

Freshly ground black pepper

2 tsp lemon juice

Method:

1. Peel and coarsely grate the carrots and potato. Finely chop the onion. Heat oil in a large pan, add the grated vegetables and onion. Cook for 5 minutes the add the stock, rice, large pinch

of nutmeg and black pepper if required.

2. Bring to the boil, and then simmer for 45 minutes. Add lemon juice and serve with more nutmeg grated on top.

Creamy Cauliflower Soup

Serves 4 - 6

Ingredients:

2 medium potatoes, scrubbed and chopped

2 cups / 500ml milk substitute

2 cups / 500ml vegetable stock

Sea salt

I medium cauliflower, cut into small pieces

Handful of fresh mint leaves or 2 tsp dried mint

1 tsp ground nutmeg

1 tsp ground black pepper

Method:

1. Simmer together the potatoes, milk, stock and salt, gently in a large pan until the potatoes are really soft.

2. Add the rest of the ingredients to the pan and simmer uncovered for approximately 20 minutes, until the cauliflower is tender.

3. Let cool slightly and blend until smooth - not for too long or the potato can become gluey. Serve.

Courgette and Tarragon Soup

This soup is delicious and more filling than you would expect

Serves 4- 6

Ingredients:

1 large onion, chopped

3 tbs olive oil

6 to 8 medium courgettes, roughly chopped

3 tbs dried or fresh tarragon leaves

1 ½ cups / 400ml milk substitute to taste –

if too thick add more milk

2 cups / 500ml vegetable stock

Sea salt

1 tsp ground black pepper

Method:

1. Sauté the onion in the oil gently until soft, but do not let go brown. Add the courgettes and herbs and stir.

2. Add the rest of the ingredients, except milk substitute, bring to the boil, reduce heat and simmer gently for 10 to 15 minutes. Add milk and bring to simmer for 5 minutes, let soup cool a little, then blend in a food processor or blender until smooth.

Watercress Soup

Serves 4 - 6

Ingredients: 2 bunches of watercress

850ml vegetable stock

1 tbs fresh parsley chopped

1 tbs fresh mint leaves

2 tbs yoghurt substitute (optional)

Method:

1. Wash and trim the watercress, and add it to the stock, together with the parley and mint.

2. Cook gently for a few minutes, then put in a food blender, and blend briefly. Reheat and add the yoghurt just before serving.

Apple and Watercress Soup

Serves 4 -6 A chilled, tasty and nutritious soup

Ingredients:

6 eating apples, peeled, cored and sliced

1130ml vegetable stock

2 bunches watercress

Juice of 1 lemon

Sea salt

Ground black pepper

4 tbs yoghurt substitute (optional)

Method:

1. Heat the stock, add the apples, and simmer until they are soft.

2. Meanwhile, wash the watercress and trim off the stalks. Reserve enough leaves for use as a garnish and add the rest to the apple stock. Simmer for a few minutes more, then blend in a blender. Add the lemon juice, season to taste and leave to chill.

3. To serve, pour into 4 bowls, add a swirl of yoghurt to each, and a sprig of watercress.

Almond Creamy Soup

This is a great soup base for chilled, raw soups. You can also heat the soups if you prefer them hot. This soup base can be used to create numerous wonderful variations.

Ingredients:

1½ cups / 200g sprouted almonds, blanched

2 cups / 500ml filtered water

2 lemons, juiced

1 garlic clove

1 tbs. flaxseed oil

½ tsp. ground cumin

½ tsp. sea salt

freshly ground black pepper

Method:

1. See 'Almonds Sprouts' in the Tips and Techniques on how to sprout and blanche almonds.

2. Put all ingredients above into a blender and blend very well. This is your Almond Creamy Soup Base.

Try the variations below.

Lemon Courgette Bisque: Add in:

2 small courgettes, grated

½ cup / 2 to 3 spring onions - finely minced

1/3rd cup / 80ml lemon juice

Corn-of-the-Cob: Add in:

1 corn, cut off the cob

¼ cup / 1 to 2 spring onions - finely minced

¼ red bell pepper, finely chopped

2 mushrooms, finely chopped

Almond-beet Borsht: Add in:

½ beet, grated

½ cup / 60g chopped cucumber

¼ cup / 30g finely minced chives

sprinkle of chopped dill

Creamy Spinach Swirl: Add in:

½ bunch spinach

½ tsp. garam masala

Divide the soup base in half. Put one half back into the blender with spinach and garam masala and blend well. Pour the white soup base into 2 or 4 soup bowls, and then pour the green spinach blend into each bowl. With a spoon stir gently. Because of the spices, this soup will keep for 2 days in the refrigerator.

Salads

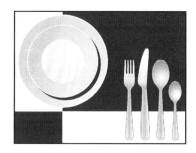

Mushroom Salad with Walnuts and Watercress

Ingredients:

Vinaigrette:

1 large spring onion, finely diced

¼ tsp salt

1 tbs red wine vinegar

2 tbs walnut or olive oil

Salad:

2 large mushrooms, stems removed

3 tbs walnut or olive oil, plus a little extra

1 bunch watercress stems discarded, washed and dried

3 tablespoons walnuts, roasted and chopped

1 tbs olive oil

Salt and pepper

Method:

1. For vinaigrette: combine spring onion, salt and vinegar in a bowl. Whisk 2 tablespoons walnut oil into mixture. Season to taste with pepper.
2. Brush mushrooms with remaining oil; sprinkle with salt and pepper. Grill for 4 minutes per side.
3. Cut mushrooms into wide strips. Toss with 1 tablespoon vinaigrette.
4. Arrange watercress and walnuts on salad plates and spoon remaining vinaigrette evenly over each. Arrange mushrooms on top.

Broad Bean and Mushroom Salad

Ingredients:

2 cups / 300g shelled, young broad beans

1 cup / 75g button mushrooms, sliced

3 - 4 spring onions, finely chopped

A big bunch of fresh parsley, washed and chopped

3 tbs olive oil

1 tsp lemon juice

2 cloves garlic, finely chopped

Salt and pepper

Method:

Put the beans, button mushrooms, and spring onions in a bowl. Pour the olive oil into the bowl and toss salad gently - being careful not to break the tender beans. Sprinkle in the lemon juice, garlic, salt and pepper. Sprinkle the parsley over the top.

Avocado, Spinach and Mushroom Salad

Ingredients:

2 cups / 60g young spinach leaves

1 cups / 75g mushrooms, cleaned and sliced

1 avocado pear

1 tbs lemon juice

2 tbs olive oil

Salt and pepper

1 tbs fresh chopped parsley

1 tbs pine nuts (optional)

Method:

1. Wash the spinach thoroughly in several changes of water, dry thoroughly and arrange in a deep bowl. Arrange the mushrooms and avocado on top of the spinach, and sprinkle with lemon juice.

2. When you are ready to serve the salad, spoon over the oil, and season to taste. Scatter on top the chopped parsley, and the pine nuts. Toss gently just before serving.

Cucumber-Avocado Salad with Toasted Cumin Dressing

Avocado mixed with vegetables and fragrant cumin dressing makes a nice change of pace from guacamole.

Ingredients:

1 tbs cumin seeds

3 tbs fresh lemon juice

1/3rd cup / 80ml mild olive oil

Sea salt and black pepper

6 cups / 300g prepared mixed salad greens

1 small avocado, peeled, cut into 1-inch cubes

1 tomato, cored, seeded, chopped

1 small cucumber, seeded and diced

2 tbs finely chopped red onion

Method:

1. **For the dressing -** In small dry pan over low heat, toast cumin seeds 2 minutes or until fragrant, stirring occasionally, and place in small bowl. Add lemon juice and whisk well. Add oil in a thin, steady stream, whisking until blended. Add salt and pepper to taste.

2. **For the salad -** In a large salad bowl, combine greens with ¼ cup/ 70ml dressing; toss to coat. Place on serving plates. Mix avocado, tomato, cucumber, and onion with remaining dressing; toss to coat. Top each portion of greens with avocado mixture.

Sweet Potato and Spinach Salad

This salad dressing is less acidic than most, allowing the orange flavour to come through. To make ahead, prep your ingredients the night before, chilling the dressing in an airtight container and the vegetables in separate sandwich bags.

Ingredients:

Dressing:

1/3rd cup / 30g very thinly sliced onion

1 tbs oil of choice (nut oil is good)

1 tbs orange juice

1½ tsp. rice wine vinegar (not sweetened or seasoned)

Sea salt to taste

Salad:

1 medium sweet potato, peeled and cut into ½ " dice

4 cups / 120g packed spinach leaves

1 small red bell pepper, cut into matchsticks

Method:

1. Combine dressing ingredients in a bowl with a whisk or fork.

2. Put potato in a small saucepan with enough water to cover and bring to a boil; cook 7 to 8 minutes until tender but not mushy. Drain in colander and rinse briefly under cold water to stop the cooking.

3. Toss dressing with potato, spinach, and pepper. Serve immediately.

This salad is chock full of vitamins and minerals. Sweet potatoes provide beta-carotene (a precursor of vitamin A), vitamin C, and potassium. Spinach contributes iron and vitamin B2.

Basmati Rice, Apple and Walnut Salad

Ingredients:

1/3rd cup / 35g walnuts

2 tbs olive oil

Zest from one orange

½ cup / 150ml orange juice

2 tbs apple cider vinegar

½ tsp sea salt

¼ tsp black pepper

¼ tsp ground nutmeg

4 cups / 1000g cooked brown basmati rice

1 apple, cut into 1/4-inch pieces

3 stalks of celery cut into ¼ -inch slices

5 or 6 pale green celery leaves, chopped

4 sprigs parsley, chopped

Method:

1. Roast the walnuts in a preheated 350ºF/180ºC oven for 5 to 7 minutes. Chop coarsely and set aside.

2. In a large bowl, combine the olive oil, orange zest, orange juice, vinegar, sea salt, pepper, and nutmeg. Mix well.

3. To this mixture, add the rice, apple, celery, and celery leaves. Also add the parsley and chopped walnuts. Toss all together until the salad is well-mixed.

Cucumber, Mango and Black Bean Salad

Mangoes and black beans are high in nutrients and fibre. This salad would make a great accompaniment to any grilled food.

Ingredients:

1 cucumber, washed and cut into ½ " dice

½ of 1 medium mango, cut into ½ " dice

½ cup / 50g drained and rinsed black beans

2 tbs fresh lime juice

2 tbs orange juice

1 tbs finely chopped fresh coriander

¾ tsp salt

1 jalapeno pepper, seeded and finely chopped

Method:

In a large bowl, toss all ingredients. Let stand 10 minutes for flavours to blend.

Beany Salad

Ingredients:

2 sticks celery

½ green pepper (bell)

1 medium tomato

2 spring onions

3 oz cucumber

Small can sweet-corn, drained and rinsed

1 cup / 60g chickpeas cooked and drained.

Method:

Wash and finely chop celery, pepper, tomato, onions and cucumber. Mix all ingredients together and toss with a dressing of your choice. (See Dressings further in the book)

A Different Chopped Salad

Just a small amount of wild rice adds a delightfully chewy texture to this easy chopped salad.

Ingredients:

2 tbs olive or vegetable oil

1 tbs red wine vinegar

¾ teaspoon sea salt

½ cup / 50g very thinly sliced red onion

1½ / 850gm pounds fresh green beans, trimmed

1 small head radicchio, coarsely chopped

¾ cup / 200g cooked wild rice (about 1/3 cup raw)

½ cup / 100g chopped tomato

Method:

1.   In a large bowl, combine oil, vinegar and salt; stir in onion and let stand until beans are ready.

2.   In lightly salted boiling water, cook green beans 7 to 8 minutes, until tender but still bright green.

Drain in a colander under cold running water; shake to drain excess moisture. Stack in bundles and cut into 1/2" pieces.

3. Place green beans, radicchio, rice and tomato in a large bowl; toss with dressing to coat.

Tangy Bean and Spinach Salad

Ingredients:

10 oz canned pinto beans, or lima beans, drained and rinsed

2/3rds cup / 300g florets cauliflower

2/3rds cup / 300g red bell pepper, chopped

¾ small avocado, peeled, pitted, and cubed

1 to 2 spring onions, with tops, sliced

1/3rd cup / 80ml dressing (see selection in Dressings)

2 ½ cups / 80g baby spinach leaves

2 tangerines, peeled a divided into segment

1 tbs. plus 1 tsp. roasted sunflower seeds, optional

Method:

1. Combine beans and vegetables in salad bowl; pour dressing over salad and toss.
2. Add spinach and oranges and toss; season to taste with salt and pepper. Spoon salad into bowls; sprinkle with sunflower seeds.

South American Salad Mix

Quinoa is a Gluten free gain. This main dish salad features quinoa, an ancient Inca grain. High-protein quinoa cooks in 15 minutes, so it's great for fast meals. This is a recipe is a meal in itself.

Ingredients:

Quinoa Salad:

1 cup / 175g quinoa, well rinsed

1 cup frozen sweet-corn kernels, thawed

 - or 1 small can of sweet-corn

Juice of one lemon

1 tbs olive oil

2 to 3 spring onions, finely chopped

Sea salt and black pepper, to taste

Bean salad:

1 16-ounce (455g) can pinto beans, drained

1 cup / 200g diced tomato

1 tbs apple cider

¼ cup / 30g chopped parsley or coriander

Freshly ground black pepper, to taste

Garnishes of pumpkin seeds and olives

Method:

1. Boil 2 cups / 500ml water in a saucepan. Add the quinoa and simmer, covered, for 15 minutes. When done, fluff with a fork and transfer to a bowl. Combine quinoa with remaining ingredients for the quinoa salad.
2. While the quinoa cooks, toss the bean salad ingredients in another bowl.

To assemble, spread quinoa salad evenly on a platter. Leave a well in the centre and mound bean salad into the well. Sprinkle with pumpkin seed and olives.

Spicy Red Beans and Rice Salad

Ingredients:

1 lb / 500gm canned red kidney beans

¾ cup / 200g cooked long grain rice

1 to 2 spring onions, sliced

2 to 3 fresh diced tomatoes

½ tsp sea salt

½ tsp garlic, finely chopped

¼ tsp cayenne pepper

1/8th tsp finely ground black pepper

¼ tsp dried basil

¼ tsp dried thyme

¼ tsp dried oregano

1½ tsp red wine vinegar

1½ tbs extra virgin olive oil

Method:

1. Using a strainer, drain beans and rinse very well, being careful to not break the beans. Transfer to flat serving dish and toss gently with rice, onions, and tomato. Set aside.

2. Make a creole spice mix in a separate bowl by combining salt, garlic salt, peppers, basil, thyme, and oregano. Stir well to combine. Sprinkle just 1 tsp. of this mix over bean mixture. Add vinegar and olive oil. Let stand 5 minutes, and then toss gently with bean mixture. Serve immediately.

Spicy Sprouted Bean Salad

Ingredients:

2 cups / 200g sprouted mung beans (or lentils)

2-4 tbs freshly grated coconut

1 ½ tbs sesame oil

1-2 tbs lemon juice

¼ tsp garam masala

1/8th tsp ground brown mustard seeds

1/8th tsp ground cumin seeds

1/8th tsp cayenne pepper (optional)

Sea salt

Method:

Put all the ingredients into a bowl and mix well together. Adjust flavours by adding more lemon juice, coconut or seasoning to taste. Keeps for 2-3 days in refrigerator.

Spicy Pasta Salad

This is a main meal salad

Ingredients:

1 lb / 450g of wheat free pasta

1/3rd cup / 80ml oil of choice

¼ cup / 70ml fresh lime juice

chilli powder to taste

2 tsp ground cumin

2 cloves garlic, crushed

small can sweet corn, drained

1 can beans of choice, rinsed and drained

½ cup / 80g green (bell) pepper, chopped

½ cup / 80g red (bell) pepper, chopped

½ cup / 25g fresh coriander, chopped

1 cup or 400gm tin of plum tomatoes

Sea salt to taste

Method:

1. Cook pasta in lightly salted water, rinse and drain and put aside.
2. In a large bowl combine oil, lime juice, chilli powder, cumin, salt and garlic. Stir in the pasta and leave to stand for flavours to blend, stirring occasionally.
3. Stir in sweet-corn, beans, red and green pepper and ½ the coriander leaves. Spoon onto a serving dish, and garnish with tomato and remaining coriander.

Carrot, Orange and Sunflower Seed Salad

Ingredients:

½ cup / 150ml apple juice

2 tbs tahini

1 tbs maple syrup

1 tbs apple cider vinegar

pinch of cinnamon

2 cups / 100g carrots, shredded

1 orange, peeled, cut into segments,

and each segment cut into three pieces

1/3rd / 50g cup currants

¼ cup / 25gm sunflower seeds

¼ cup / 10gm freshly chopped parsley

Method:

In a blender or food processor, combine the apple juice, tahini, maple syrup, vinegar, and cinnamon, and process for 1 minute or until smooth and creamy. In a bowl, place the remaining ingredients, pour the dressing over the top, and toss gently to combine. Store in the refrigerator.

Bean-sprout Salad

An excellent healthy and nutritious main meal salad

Ingredients:

2 cups / 350g red pepper, cut into thin strips

2 cups / 350g carrots, cut into thin strips

3 to 4 spring onions, sliced diagonally

2 to 4 sticks celery, sliced diagonally

1 cup / 80g mushrooms, sliced

1½ cups / 150gm mung bean sprouts, rinsed

¼ cup / 75ml olive oil

2 tsp toasted sesame oil

2 tbs tamari

2 tsp lemon juice

1 tsp garlic, minced

1 tsp ginger, minced

salt and pepper to taste

2 tbs toasted sesame seeds

Method:

In a bowl, combine all of the vegetables. In another small bowl, whisk together the olive oil, sesame oil, tamari, lemon juice, garlic, and ginger. Pour dressing over vegetables and toss lightly. Season with salt and pepper to taste and sprinkle with toasted sesame seeds.

Indian Style Sprouted Lentil Salad

Ingredients:

¼ cup / 100g dry lentils

½ cup / 80g cucumber, quartered and sliced

½ cup / 80g green pepper, diced

½ cup / 80g radishes, quartered and sliced

2 to 3 tomatoes diced

1/3rd cup / 35 gm spring onion, thinly sliced

2 tbs lemon juice

2 tbs olive oil

1 ½ tsp dried oregano

1 tsp curry powder

½ tsp dry mustard

Method:

1. Begin by soaking and sprouting the lentils (see Sprouting Seeds) It should take 3-5 days for the lentils to sprout 1-2-inch long tails. Then place the sprouted lentils in indirect sunlight for several-hours to create chlorophyll and to turn the sprouted tails green before using. Using 1/4 cups dry lentils should yield 4 cups sprouted lentils.

2. Carefully rinse the sprouted lentils in a colander to remove any of the loose hulls- the hulls should sink to the bottom of the colander as you rinse- then transfer the sprouted lentils to a bowl and discard the loosened hulls.

3. Add the chopped vegetables to the bowl and lightly toss them with the sprouted lentils. In a

72

small bowl, whisk together the remaining ingredients. Drizzle the dressing over the vegetable mixture and toss gently again. Allow the flavours to blend for 20-30 minutes before serving.

This crunchy salad also makes an excellent sandwich or filling.

Warm Cauliflower Salad

Serves 4 -6

Ingredients:

1 cauliflower, divided into florets, stalks and leaves shredded

Juice of 1 lemon

2 tsp cider vinegar

2 tbs chopped fresh parsley

1 tbs chopped fresh mint

1 tbs light tahini

1 tsp ground black pepper

Method:
1. Cook the cauliflower in boiling water for about 7 minutes, drain and put into a warm serving dish.
2. Whisk all the other ingredients together. Pour over the warm cauliflower and serve at once.

Tunisian Style Carrot Salad

Serves 4 - 6

Ingredients:

½ cup / 150ml oil

2 garlic cloves, very thinly sliced

1 lb / 450g carrots, scrubbed and cut into thin strips

2 tbs cider vinegar

4 spring onions, sliced

½ tsp ground cloves

½ tsp ground cumin seeds

½ tsp paprika

1 tsp tamari

Method:
1. Heat the oil and toss in the carrots and garlic. Let sizzle for 2 minutes. Reduce the heat, cover and cook for 3 - 5 minutes more.
2. Add the rest of the ingredients to the pan - in the order of the list above - stir well, then remove from the heat.
3. Transfer to a bowl and chill before serving.

Mediterranean Carrot Salad

Ingredients:

Juice and grated rind of 1 orange

Juice and grated rind of 1 lemon

2 tbs olive oil

Fresh ground pepper

Sea salt

1 lb / 450g carrots

1 tbs pine nuts

1 tbs raisins

Method:

1. Scrub the orange and lemon carefully before grating their rinds into a bowl. Add their juices and the oil, then season with a little salt and pepper. Mix well.

2. Peel and grate the carrots. Put them in a dish and add the dressing, the pine nuts and raisins. Toss well, and leave to stand for an hour or more in a cool place before serving

Salad Suedoise

Serves 4 - 6

Ingredients:

Dressing:

4 tbs olive oil

4 tbs cider vinegar

2 tsp yellow mustard seeds,

 (soaked overnight in cider vinegar)

1 tsp fresh dill, finely chopped

1 tbs light tahini

1 tbs tamari

1 tsp ground black pepper

Vegetables:

4 medium courgettes, grated

2 apples, grated

2 carrots, grated

4 celery sticks, finely chopped

Method:

1. Make up the dressing by mixing all ingredients in a blender

2. Gently fold the vegetables into the dressing and serve.

This dressing also works well with cooked potatoes and butter beans. Try a few experiments yourself. Serve with a green salad and home-made bread.

Oriental Aubergine Salad

Serves 4 - 6

Ingredients:

½ cup / 150ml olive oil

2 aubergines cut into ½ inch slices

2 onions, thinly sliced

Ground black pepper

2 tbs fresh coriander, chopped

2 tbs fresh dill leaves, chopped

Splash of cider vinegar

Squeeze of lemon juice

Method:

1. Generously oil a baking sheet and spread a single layer of aubergine slices on it. Cover with a layer of onion and a sprinkling of oil and black pepper. (You may need to cook in 2 batches due to the amount) Bake in the oven for about 40 minutes at 475°F/250°C. Cool and chop roughly

2. Stir the remaining ingredients into the aubergines. Chill and serve. Nice with hot bread – wheat free

Mediterranean Rice Salad

Serves 4 - 6

Ingredients:

2 cups / 500ml cooked brown rice i.e. 1 cup raw rice

20 black olives, stoned and halved

4 ripe tomatoes, chopped

Kernels cut from 2 cooked corn cobs or

1 small can of sweet corn

Handful of fresh basil, chopped

3 garlic cloves, crushed

2 tbs olive oil

2 tbs tamari

Juice and zest of 1 lemon

1 red (bell) pepper finely chopped

Method:

Mix all ingredients gently together. Leave to stand for 1 hour before serving.

Middle Eastern Rice Salad

Serves 4 – 6

Ingredients:

2 cups / 500ml brown rice, cooked i.e 1 cup raw rice

6 chopped dates, fresh or dried

3 tbs toasted cashew nuts

4 spring onions, finely sliced

2 tbs tamari

1 tsp toasted fennel seeds

1 tsp toasted cumin seeds

Juice of 1 lemon

3 tbs olive oil

Method:

Gently mix all ingredients together and set to one side to 'develop' before serving.

Brown Rice Salad

Serves 4 - 6

Ingredients:

2 cups / 500ml brown rice

3 spring onions finely chopped

1 red pepper (bell pepper) chopped

2 oz / 50g raisins

2oz / 50g cashews, roasted and chopped

Salt and pepper

Method:

Cook rice, rinse, drain and cool. Place in a bowl and add other ingredients. Add salad dressing of choice

Toss and serve

The Vegetable Selection

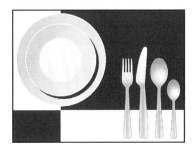

Some of these dishes in the first section can be meals in themselves by adding rice, wheat free pasta, wheat free breads. Try adding some of the sauces from the Sauces collection. Otherwise these dishes can be used to accompany chicken or fish for your main meal.

Vegetable Tabbouleh – not the couscous version

Ingredients:

1 bunch cauliflower

3 tbs olive oil

1 tsp curry powder

2 bunches parsley

8-10 leaves fresh mint (optional)

1 medium onion

1 large cucumber

2 medium tomatoes

1/3rd cup / 30ml fresh lemon juice

¼ tsp salt

¼ tsp garlic powder or fresh garlic

1. **Method:**
    Cut cauliflower florets into uniform pieces. Put cauliflower into food processor and pulse to grate into uniform granules, about 1 minute.
2. Heat 1 tablespoon of the oil in a 12-inch non-stick skillet or wok over medium-high heat. Add curry powder and cook until it sizzles slightly but does not burn. Add grated cauliflower and stir fry, turn until it is cooked, about 10 minutes. Remove from heat and cool.
3. Meanwhile, rinse parsley and mint and trim and discard large stems. Chop into very small pieces.
4. In a large bowl combine reserved cooked cauliflower, parsley, onion, cucumber and tomato.
5. In a small bowl mix remaining 2 tablespoons olive oil, lemon juice, & salt. Pour over cauliflower mixture and toss to mix well. Serve at room temp or on chilled Romaine lettuce leaves.

Ginger, Almond and Garlic Broccoli

The ginger-garlic duo livens up the flavour of broccoli, and a crunch of almonds adds the finishing touch.

Ingredients:

2 tbs olive oil

2 tbs finely sliced peeled fresh ginger-root

2 tbs slivered almonds

2 garlic cloves, thinly sliced

1 bunch broccoli, cut into 1" florets, stems peeled and cut into ¼ "thick slices

¼ cup / 70ml vegetable stock

1 tablespoon white wine vinegar

Method:

1. In a large heavy skillet or wok, heat oil over medium-high heat. Cook ginger, almonds and garlic until golden, about 3 minutes. With a slotted spoon, transfer mixture to a paper towel to drain.

2. Add broccoli to skillet and cook until crisp-tender, about 5 minutes. Stir in stock and vinegar. Bring to a boil, and cook until liquid is almost evaporated. Toss the broccoli with ginger mixture before serving.

Grilled Peppers and Onions

Grilling vegetables seems to bring out their flavour. In this recipe, peppers and onions are tossed with tangy olive vinaigrette.

Ingredients:

2 medium bell peppers, cut in half and seeded

2 small onions cut in ½ " thick slices

3 tbs olive oil

1 tbs balsamic vinegar

2 tbs pitted oil-cured black olives

1 tsp capers, drained

Salt and pepper

Method:

Prepare a medium grill.

1. Cook vegetables 4 to 5 minutes per side until peppers are blistered and onions are nicely browned. Remove from grill; cool 5 minutes.

2. In a medium bowl mix olive oil, vinegar, olives and capers. Cut pepper into 1/2" strips and onions into 1/2" pieces. Add vegetables to bowl. Toss gently to combine ingredients. Season to taste with salt and pepper.

Grilled Green and Yellow Squash with Basil

Grilling adds a smoky flavour which enhances the delicate flavour of mild vegetables, like squash. Fresh basil and an accent of lemon juice are all that is needed to finish this dish.

Ingredients:

2 medium courgettes, trimmed and cut diagonally into ¼ " slices

1 medium yellow squash, trimmed and cut diagonally into ¼ " slices

2 tbs olive oil

½ tsp salt

¼ tsp pepper

3 tbs thinly sliced basil leaves

1 tbs chopped fresh parsley

2 tsp fresh lemon juice

½ tsp grated lemon rind

1 tbs liquid sweetener (like Amsake or Rice Syrup)

Method:

1. Prepare a medium grill. In a large bowl, combine courgettes, yellow squash, oil, salt and pepper. Toss to coat.

2. Grill squash (in batches, if necessary) 2 to 3 minutes per side until lightly charred and just tender. Transfer to a large bowl and toss with basil, parsley, lemon juice, lemon rind and liquid sweetener.

Sesame Broccoli, Red Pepper and Spinach

A trio of vegetables is flavoured Asian-style, with sesame, garlic, and hot pepper.

Ingredients:

1 tbs sesame seeds

1 tsp olive oil

1 bunch broccoli, cut into 1-inch florets, stems peeled and cut into 2" x ¼ " strips

1 red bell pepper, cut into thin strips

1 garlic clove, finely chopped

10 oz / 300g washed spinach

1 small hot red chilli or jalapeño pepper, seeded, finely chopped

2 tsp sesame oil

Method:

1. Toast sesame seeds in a large non-stick skillet over medium heat, stirring until golden brown and fragrant. Transfer to a small bowl.

2. Heat oil over medium heat in same pan until hot. Add broccoli and red pepper; cook until broccoli is crisp-tender, about 5 minutes. Add garlic, spinach, jalapeño, and sesame oil, mix well.

3. Cover and cook until spinach is wilted, about 2 minutes. Sprinkle with toasted sesame seeds.

Spinach and Cannellini Beans

This hearty meal can be made with almost any dried bean, such as Black-eye beans, Haricot or Chick-peas.

Ingredients:

8 oz / 220g cannellini beans, soaked overnight

4 tbs olive oil

1 onion, chopped

3 - 4 tomatoes, peeled and chopped

½ tsp paprika

1 lb / 450g spinach

2 garlic cloves, chopped

Sea salt to taste

Freshly ground black pepper

Method:

1. Drain the beans, place in a saucepan and cover with water. Bring to boil and boil rapidly for 10 minutes. Cover and simmer for about 1 hour until they are tender.

2. Fry the onion and garlic in 1 tbs of the oil over a gentle heat until soft but not brown, then add

the tomatoes and continue cooking over a gentle heat.

3.   Heat the remaining oil in a large pan, stir in the paprika and then add the spinach. Cover and cook for a few minutes until the spinach has wilted.

4.   Add the onion and tomato mixture to the spinach, mix well and stir in the cannellini beans adding salt and pepper to taste. Serve with fresh wheat-free bread as a main meal.

Ratatouille

Ratatouille is a French vegetable casserole which became well known in the States in the 1970's. Great as a side dish, can be served with baked potatoes and salad for a main meal, or used as a topping for a pasta dish (using non wheat based pasta)

Ingredients:

1 small aubergine (about 1 ½ pounds / 500g), cut into 1" pieces

1/3rd cup / 80ml olive oil

4 garlic cloves, pushed through a press or finely chopped

1 tsp salt

½ tsp dried rosemary

½ tsp dried thyme

¼ tsp black pepper

1 medium courgette, cut into 1" pieces

1 yellow squash, cut into 1" pieces

1 small red pepper, cut into 1/2" pieces

1 small tomato, cut into 1/2" pieces

1 small onion, thinly sliced

Method:

1.   Sprinkle aubergine with salt; place in a colander and let bitter juices drain 20 minutes. Rinse eggplant and pat dry.

2.   Heat oven to 425° F / 220c. In a 10 x 15 baking dish, mix oil, garlic, salt, rosemary, thyme, and pepper. Add vegetables, toss to coat evenly with oil mixture.

3.   Cover dish with foil and bake 15 minutes. Uncover and cook 30 minutes more, mixing occasionally, until vegetables are tender and browned.

Baked Courgettes

Serves 4

Ingredients:

4 small to medium courgettes

6 - 8 tomatoes, chopped

1 clove garlic, crushed

Pinch of oregano

Pinch of basil

¼ tsp paprika

Method:

Preheat oven to 375°F/190°C.

1.   Cut the courgettes in half lengthways and scoop out the soft centre part, then arrange them on a baking dish.

2.   Mix all the other ingredients together, add the scooped-out courgette, and pour over the cour-

gette 'boats', filling the boat-shapes and allowing to overflow. Bake for 30 minutes.

Nut Mince

If you want to make a meal that requires savoury mince, for example, Shepherd's Pie, Spaghetti Bolognaise, Mince Pie etc., then try this alternative mix. It has a nice texture and tastes good.

Serves 4

Ingredients:

1 large onion

½ tbs basil

1 tbs olive oil

14 oz / 400g can tomatoes

8oz / 225g finely ground walnuts or hazelnuts

4 oz / 110g non wheat breadcrumbs

2 tbs chutney

Salt and pepper

Method:

1. Fry onion with herbs until brown

2. Add tomatoes and all other ingredients. Cook gently for 20 minutes

You can add finely chopped carrots or celery if in season. You can always add more spices and herbs to this basic recipe

Spicy Oven Fries

Try serving these with soup for a delicious change to the usual bread.

Serves 4 - 6

Ingredients:

2 tbs olive oil

1 tbs tomato puree

1 tsp paprika

1 tbs tamari

1 tsp ground black pepper

3 to 4 large potatoes, scrubbed and cut into fairly fat 'fingers'

Method:

1. Whisk together the spices, pepper and oil in a large mixing bowl

2. Toss the potato fingers in the mixture, making sure they are evenly covered. Turn into a roasting tin and bake for 35 - 40 minutes, until soft in the middle and a bit crunchy around the edges.

Courgette and Potato Rosti

Serves 4 - 6

Ingredients:

3 medium potatoes, skins left on, scrubbed and coarsely grated

1 courgette, grated

1 tsp ground black pepper

1 tsp black poppy seeds

Pinch of fresh thyme leaves

1 tbs rice flour

3 tbs olive oil

Method:

1. Mix all ingredients together well, except the oil. Leave for 10 minutes before squeezing the liquid out firmly - twisting the mixture in a clean tea-towel is quite effective.

2. Heat the oil in a heavy frying pan. Put the potato mixture in the pan and press gently to an even thickness. Cook gently without stirring or covering for 20 minutes.

3. Turn the rosti over. This is considerably easier if you have another oiled pan to place over the top and invert the whole thing carefully into this other pan - but this is rather a heavy operation. Alternatively, use an oiled plate and slide the turned rosti back into the same pan. Cook gently for 15 - 20 minutes more. Serve at once.

This can be turned into a tasty and filling dish by adding a pouring sauce (see sauces) of your choice, to pour over the rosti, and a salad or other vegetable dish of choice.

Parsnip and Carrots with Sesame and Maple Glaze

Serves 4 - 6

Ingredients:

Oven 375 F / 190c.

2 good sized parsnips, scrubbed and cubed

4 carrots, scrubbed and cubed

2 tbs sesame seeds

2 tbs olive oil

2 tbs maple syrup

1 tsp tamari (optional)

Zest and juice of ½ an orange

Method:

Oven 375 F / 190C.

1. Cook carrots in water for about 5 minutes. Add the parsnips and boil for a further 5 minutes. Drain.

2. Mix together the olive oil, sesame seeds, maple syrup and orange rind and juice in a bowl. Gently stir in the carrots and parsnips to coat. Turn into a roasting tin and bake in the oven for 20 to 25 minutes, until just browning

Grilled Aubergines with Salsa Verde

Serves 4 - 6

Ingredients:

2 medium aubergines

- cut lengthways into ½ inch slices

2 large tomatoes, finely chopped

4 tbs olive oil

2 garlic cloves, peeled and roughly chopped

2 tbs parsley

2 tbs fresh basil

2 tbs pine nuts or almonds

½ tsp ground black pepper

½ cup / 140ml olive oil

Method:

1. Brush the aubergine slices with a little oil and grill on both sides until golden brown and soft (about 10 minutes)

2. Mix all the other ingredients, except tomatoes, in a blender and process to a smoothish paste

3. Layer the aubergine slices alternately with the tomatoes. Pour over the salsa and serve.

Nice served just warm or chilled with hot bread or rice to make it into a main meal.

Ginger and Sesame Carrots

This dish is full of goodness with the ginger and garlic added to the carrots.

Serves 4- 6

Ingredients:

3 tbs olive oil

¼ cup sesame seeds

¼ cup / 70ml fresh root ginger, peeled and grated

2 garlic cloves, grated

6 medium carrots, scrubbed and cut into match-sticks or thin diagonal slices.

Method:

Heat the oil and sesame seeds together in a wok or an enamelled iron casserole. When the seeds begin to pop, add the ginger, garlic and stir. Add the carrots and stir well. Lower the heat a little, cover and cook for 6 - 10 minutes, stirring once during this time. Serve immediately.

Spicy Lentil and Rice Mix

This savoury mix of lentils, fragrant basmati rice, garlic, caramelised onions, and raisins makes a ter-rific main dish with a salad, or side dish.

Ingredients:

3 cups / 675g basmati rice

8–10 cups / 2000ml water

1½ cups / 300g lentils

8 cups / 2000ml water

4 tbs oil

2 tsp sea salt

¼ tsp saffron

2 onions, thinly sliced

2 cloves of garlic, chopped

3 tbs oil

1 cup / 150g raisins

½ tsp cinnamon

½ tsp turmeric

½ tsp cumin

½ tsp sea salt

¼ tsp pepper

Method:

1. Wash lentils thoroughly, add water to a medium-sized pot and boil uncovered on medium-high for 10–15 minutes or until done (don't overcook). Drain lentils in a colander, saving the liquid. Dissolve the saffron in a small amount of hot water and add to the lentils. Set aside.

2. Wash the rice thoroughly. To a separate pot add water, half of the oil and salt and bring to a boil. On high heat, boil the rice for about 10 to 15 minutes or until slightly soft. Drain rice in a large colander and rinse with warm water.

3. In a large heavy-bottom pot, coat the bottom of the pot with the remaining oil and add 1/3 of the rice. Add 1/3 of the lentils and mix well. Repeat until all the rice and lentils are mixed in the pot.

4. Shape the rice/lentil mixture into a pyramid and cover with a lid and steam over a medium to medium-low heat for about 30 to 40 minutes.

5. Slice the onions thinly and lightly brown over low heat with oil. Add the remaining ingredients and cook for about 5 more minutes. Serve the lentil rice on a serving platter and top off with the caramelised onion mixture.

Main Dishes

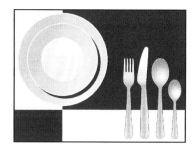

Mung Bean and Sage Cottage Pie

Serves 4 - 6

Ingredients:

1 lb / 450g mung beans or aduki beans

3 lbs / 1350g potatoes, scrubbed

2 onions, finely chopped

2 carrots, grated

2/3 tbs fresh sage leaves

½ pint / 300ml milk substitute

6 garlic cloves

½ cup / 60g corn flour

1 cup/ 250ml apple juice

2 cups / 500ml water of cooking liquid from beans

½ cup / 150ml tamari

5 tbs olive oil

1 tsp ground black pepper

Sea salt

Method:

1. Cook the beans for 45 minutes in boiling water, to which the garlic cloves have been added. Reserve the water for later use in this recipe if desired.

2. Boil potatoes with their skins on until they are tender. Then drain and mash well, adding the milk and oil.

3. Mix the corn-flour to a smooth paste with a little liquid, the carefully mix in apple juice and tamari.

4. Sauté together the onion, sage, carrots and pepper in olive oil, until soft, about 10 - 15 minutes. Add the mung beans, stir well and pour in the apple juice mixture and simmer, stirring until thickened. Tip into a greased oven-proof dish, top with the mashed potato and bake for about 20 minutes, at 425°F/220°C, until just browned.

Vegetable Goulash

Serves 6

Ingredients:

2 cups / 300g onion, diced

2 cups / 300g carrot, diced

2 cups / 350g courgettes, diced

2 tbs olive oil

2 tbs tomato paste

2 tbs Hungarian paprika

2 tbs freshly chopped parsley

¼ tsp ground nutmeg

2 cups / 400g tomatoes diced

1 - 15 oz. can kidney beans, rinsed and drained

1 - 15 oz. can cannellini beans (or other white bean)

1 cup / 250ml tomato juice

1 tsp sea salt

¼ tsp freshly ground black pepper

yoghurt to garnish

Method:

1. In a large pot, gently cook the onion, carrot, and courgette in the olive oil, for 5-7 minutes or until soft. Add the tomato paste, paprika, parsley, and nutmeg, and cook an additional 2 minutes.

2. Add the remaining ingredients, reduce the heat to low, and simmer for 15 minutes. Taste and adjust the seasonings, if needed. Serve the goulash in bowls alone, or over pasta, grains, or mashed potatoes.

This is a good recipe for bulk cooking, to freeze some for another day.

Cassoulet

Cassoulet, a hearty white bean casserole, is a French original. Its savoury flavour comes from herbes de Provence, a mixture of dried thyme, basil, rosemary and lavender.

Ingredients:

Cassoulet base:

2 tbs olive oil

1 medium onion, diced

1 large carrot, diced

1 large red potato, diced

6 large cloves garlic, minced

1 tbs herbes de Provence (or ad lib. If you cannot get hold of this mixture)

½ tsp sea salt

½ tsp freshly ground black pepper

1 bay leaf

2 x 15 oz / 420g cans cannellini beans, drained

1 x 14oz / 400g can diced tomatoes

2 cups / 500ml vegetable broth

Bread Crumb Topping:

2 tbs olive oil

3 thick slices bread (wheat-free)

2 sprigs parsley

4 cloves garlic, peeled

Preheat oven to 325°F /165°C

Method:

1. In a large pan, gently cook onion, carrot and potato in olive oil over medium heat 5 minutes. Add garlic, herbes de Provence, salt, and pepper; and cook another minute.

2. Combine vegetables with bay leaf, beans, tomatoes and vegetable broth in a large, lightly oiled casserole dish. Bake uncovered 20 minutes.

3. To make bread crumb topping, combine olive oil, bread, parsley and garlic in a food processor; puree on high until finely crumbled.

4. Remove cassoulet from oven and take out bay leaf. Raise oven temperature to 400°F (205°C). Sprinkle half the bread crumbs on top; bake another 15 minutes.

5. Remove cassoulet from oven; stir bread crumb topping into beans. Top with remaining bread crumbs. Bake another 15 minutes or until topping is lightly browned. Serve immediately.

Roasted Vegetables

These flavourful vegetables are a meal by themselves or can be served as a side dish. Leftovers are great either warm or cold.

Ingredients:

1½ lbs/ 675g potatoes, red or yellow varieties – cut into 2-inch (5cm) pieces

2 carrots, cut into 2-inch (5cm) pieces

4 spring onions, peeled and halved

8 garlic cloves, divided, minced

2 tbs olive oil, divided

1 tsp marjoram

½ lb / 225g green beans, whole

1 red pepper, cut into 2-inch (5cm) pieces

1 courgette, cut into 2-inch (5cm) chunks

½ lb / 225g mushrooms

½ tsp Sea salt

½ tsp freshly ground black pepper

Method:

Preheat oven to 375°F/190°C

1. Place potatoes, carrots, shallots and half of the minced garlic in a bowl and drizzle with 1 tbs olive oil. Toss oil and vegetables, add marjoram and mix well.

2. Spray two baking sheets with vegetable oil spray, divide and layer vegetables evenly on sheets. Place baking sheets in oven for 30 minutes.

3. While potatoes and carrots are cooking. Wash and dry remaining vegetables. Cut red pepper and courgette into 2-inch (5cm) pieces. Place vegetables in a bowl with clean mushrooms and drizzle with 1 tbs olive oil, add remaining garlic and toss gently until blended.

4. After potatoes and carrots have cooked for 30 minutes, remove from oven. Divide the green bean vegetable mixture between the two baking sheets. Mix vegetables with potatoes and carrots, forming a single layer on the baking sheet. Return to oven for another 15–20 minutes, cooking until tender.

Experiment with this recipe and try seasonal vegetables such as eggplant, yellow squash, turnips, broccoli and cauliflower.

Braised Squash with Green Lentils

Serves 4 - 6

Ingredients:

½ cup / 100g whole green lentils

2 tbs olive oil

10 spring onions chopped into 1inch lengths

2 garlic cloves, peeled and sliced

Sprig of fresh thyme

2 bay leaves

1 tsp ground black pepper

1½ lbs / 675g yellow-fleshed squash, cut into bite-size pieces, seeds and fibres removed

1 lb / 450g fresh tomatoes, finely chopped or 14oz tin chopped tomatoes

1 tbs tamari

Juice of 1 lemon

Method:

1. Cook the lentils in water or vegetable stock for 40 - 45 mins until soft. Drain and put aside.
2. Heat the oil in a pan, soften the onions and garlic with the herbs and seasoning. Add the squash. Stir, mix together and cook gently for 6 - 7 mins. Add the cooked lentils and stir gently.
3. Add tomatoes, tamari and lemon juice to pan and cook very gently for another 20 minutes, stir-ring occasionally. The dish should be soft and moist, but not runny, so allow some of the liquid to evaporate.

Serve with warm bread or rice

Lentil Bolognaise Sauce

Serves 4

Ingredients:

1 medium onion, sliced

1 stick celery, chopped

½ green pepper (bell), de-seeded and chopped

1 tbs olive oil

1 cup / 200g brown lentils

1 cup / 200g chopped tomatoes

2 bay leaves

1 tsp cinnamon

1 tsp mixed herbs

Water

Method:

1. In a large saucepan, soften the onion, celery and pepper in the oil over a low heat for 2 min-utes.
2. Rinse the lentils and add lentils, tomatoes and other ingredients to the saucepan and add suf-ficient water to cover. Bring to the boil, then put a lid on the pan and simmer over a low heat for 20 - 30 minutes, adding more water if necessary. Serve with wheat-free pasta.

Lentil Burgers

Ingredients:

1 cup / 200g red lentils

2 ½ cups / 650ml water

2 large carrots, grated

1 large onion, shopped

4 tbs rice flour

1 tsp mixed herbs

Freshly grated nutmeg

Freshly ground black pepper

Method:

Preheat oven to 400°F/200°C

1. Rinse the lentils, then place in a saucepan, cover with water and bring to the boil. Put lid on pan, reduce the heat and simmer gently till lentils are cooked and water absorbed (15 - 20 minutes). Leave to cool.

2. Put lentils into a bowl, add all other ingredients, and mix well. Shape into 8 burgers, put on floured baking tray and bake for 15 - 20 minutes.

Creamy Leek and Mushroom Croustade

Serves 4 - 6

Ingredients:

For the base:

3 tbs olive oil

2 cups / 100g soft brown bread-crumbs (wheat-free)

2/3rds cup / 120g ground hazelnuts

2/3rds cup / 120g finely chopped almonds

1 tsp tarragon

2 garlic cloves, crushed

For the filling:

2 leeks, finely chopped

1 cup / 75g sliced mushrooms

3 tbs olive oil

1 tsp ground black pepper

1 tsp ground nutmeg

½ cup / 65g wholemeal rice flour

1 cup/ 250ml nut milk

1 tbs tamari

Method:

1. To make the base - Mix all ingredients together. Press into a greased ovenproof cake tin or flan dish. Use the back of a spoon to press it down firmly. Bake for 15 minutes.

2. For the filling: Sauté the leeks and mushrooms in the oil with the pepper and nutmeg. Cover and cook over a low heat for 10 minutes. Stir in the flour and slowly add the milk, stirring all the time. Simmer gently to thicken. Spoon the mixture onto the croustade base. Splash the top with a little olive oil and tamari and return to the oven for about 10 minutes.

Serve hot with rice and vegetables or with a green salad.

Potato and Mushroom Casserole

Ingredients:

1 lb / 450g potatoes

8 oz / 225g mushrooms

2 tbs olive oil

2 cloves garlic, finely chopped

Sea salt

Fresh ground black pepper

¼ pint / 140ml yoghurt substitute

Method:

Preheat oven to 350°F/180°C

1. Peel and slice the potatoes thinly. Wipe and finely slice the mushrooms. Use half the oil to grease a fairly shallow, oven proof casserole.

2. Arrange the potatoes and mushrooms in alternating layers, finishing with a layer of potatoes. Lightly season each layer, scatter the garlic and a drizzle of yoghurt over as you build up layers. Pour the rest of the oil over the top, cover with foil and bake in the oven for about 1 ½ hours.

3. When the casserole has been cooking for about an hour, remove the foil so that the top can brown a bit. Check to see if potatoes are cooked at end of time. Cook a bit longer if required. Serve immediately.

You can add your own choice of herbs to this dish to zing it up a bit. Also try using other oils for the cooking, like nut oils to add a bit of flavour.

Full of Beans Casserole

Ingredients:

2 oz / 50g dried butter beans, soaked overnight

2 oz / 50g dried red kidney beans, soaked overnight

1 tbs olive oil

1 large onion, finely chopped

2 cloves garlic, finely chopped

2 large carrots, sliced

2 courgettes, sliced

2 celery sticks, sliced

7 oz / 200g can chopped tomatoes or fresh chopped tomatoes

1 small sprig of fresh thyme or dried thyme

Salt and pepper

Method:

1. Drain the beans, put in separate pans and cover with plenty of cold water. Bring to the boil and boil rapidly for 10 minutes, then turn the heat down, cover, and simmer for about an hour, or until the beans are tender. (This process can be speeded up if you have a pressure cooker - follow the manufacturer's instructions.)

2. Heat the oil in a heavy pan, add the onion, garlic, and let soften for a few minutes. Add the carrots, courgettes, celery, tomatoes, thyme and seasoning to taste. Add enough water to moisten.

3. Cover and simmer for about 15 minutes, adding more water if necessary, until all the vegetables are soft. Add the beans, and more water as needed. Cover, heat gently, and serve.

You can add other herbs and spices to this dish to your taste.

Creamy Golden Casserole

Serves 4 -6

Ingredients:

1 cup / 200g yellow split peas

2 cups / 500ml water or vegetable stock

6 cups / 750g yellow or orange fleshed squash - de-seeded and thickly sliced

2 tbs tamari

½ cup / 150ml coconut cream / thick coconut milk

1 cup/ 250ml boiling water

2 tbs olive oil

2 tsp black mustard seeds

Bay leaf

1 onion, sliced

1 tsp turmeric

Method:

1. Gently cook split peas in water or vegetable stock until soft. Check the pan from time to time to ensure that they do not dry out before they are cooked.

2. Mix the squash, tamari, and coconut cream with the split peas in a large casserole dish.

3. Heat the oil in a small, heavy based pan. Add the mustard seeds and stir at arm's length until they stop popping. Add the bay leaf and onion and soften for 10 minutes. Stir in the turmeric, cook for a few minutes, and tip onto squash mixture. Give it a stir, cover and bake for approximately 35 - 40 minutes, until the squash is soft.

Ideally serve with rice or chapattis made from chick-pea flour (chick-pea flour is *Gluten free*)

Barley and Mushroom Casserole

Serves 4

Ingredients:

Outer stalks and leaves of a big -

bunch celery, chopped

1 large onion, chopped

1 bunch parsley stalks

1 ½/ 850ml pints water

2 tbs olive oil

½ cup / 75g onion, finely chopped

2 cups / 200g mushrooms, finely sliced

8 oz / 225g pot barley - rinsed

½ tsp dried marjoram

½ tsp ground black pepper

Sea salt to taste

Method:

1. Make a stock with the celery, onion, parsley and water. Bring to the boil in a pan and simmer for half an hour. Cool a bit then blend in a blender.

2. Heat the oil in a heavy pan. Cook the onions and mushrooms for a few minutes, then stir in the

barley and cook until the barley begins to absorb pan juices.

3. Add the marjoram, celery stock and seasoning, bring to the boil, and simmer for 20 minutes.

4. When the barley is tender, remove the pan from the heat, transfer to a serving dish and serve.

Courgette and Bean Casserole

Serves 4 - 6

Ingredients:

3 -4 medium courgettes, washed and roughly sliced

2 cups / 400g chickpeas or bartoli beans or beans of your choice

1 medium red (bell) pepper, chopped

2 tbs olive oil

1 green (bell) pepper, chopped

3 cups / 600g chopped plumb tomatoes

2 tbs tomato puree

½ tsp cumin seeds

½ tsp coriander seeds, roughly ground in pestle and mortar

¼ tsp fenugreek seeds

1 tsp dried oregano

Sea salt

½ tsp ground black pepper

1 tsp paprika

Method:

1. Wash and soak beans overnight in water. Rinse and cook according to instructions on packet (depending on which bean you use). Drain and put aside.

2. Meanwhile, put oil in a large pan, and cook all spices at medium, heat for 3 to 4 minutes. Add the onions and cook for 4 to 5 minutes until soft, then add the red and green peppers, cook until soft.

3. Then add the courgettes, cook gently for 5 to 6 minutes. Then add puree, chopped tomatoes, salt and pepper, paprika and simmer for a further 10 minutes.

4. Add the beans and continue to cook on a low heat for about 15 to 20 minutes to allow all the flavours to blend together. Add more liquid if required i.e. vegetable stock. I make this dish quite liquid and juicy. Serve with boiled rice.

You can add a bit of chilli powder to give this dish a bit more 'kick', especially for the winter.

Arabian Stuffed Aubergines

Serves 4

Ingredients:

2 medium aubergines good and firm

6 tbs olive oil

4 cloves

2 bay leaves

1 cinnamon stick

1 medium onion. Finely chopped

4 garlic cloves, finely sliced

2 tbs tomato puree

2 tomatoes, finely chopped

½ cup / 50g pine nuts

½ tsp ground black pepper

2 tbs tamari

½ cup / 30g chopped fresh coriander

Method:

1. Drop the whole aubergines into a large pan of boiling water, boil gently for 15 minutes. Drain and cool. Cut in half length ways. Carefully cut out the flesh into pieces, keeping the skin whole.

2. Heat 4 tbs oil in a heavy based pan with the cloves, bay leaves and cinnamon. Add the onion, garlic, and soften for a few minutes. Add the tomato puree and cook for a few more minutes. Then add the tomatoes, pine nuts, pepper and tamari, along with the aubergine. Cook and stir for 5 minutes.

3. Stir in the fresh herbs and pile into the aubergine skins. Place in a greased oven-proof dish. Drizzle with a little oil and bake for 20 - 30 minutes at 350°F/180°C. Serve with rice and salad

Bean and Courgette Pie

Ingredients:

1 batch of pastry - see Baking Section

2 medium onions, sliced

1 clove garlic, crushed

6 cups / 1000g courgettes, sliced

1 tbs olive oil

6 tomatoes, skinned and chopped

1 tbs tomato puree

Herbs and spices to taste

8 oz / 225g - dried weight (any type beans,

soaked and cooked)

Method:

Preheat oven to 400°F/200°C

1. Prepare the pastry.

2. Cook onions, garlic and courgettes in the oil over a low heat for 10 minutes. Add the tomatoes, tomato puree and seasonings, cover and simmer for 5 minutes. Add the cooked beans and stir.

3. Line a flan tin with pastry, add the bean and vegetable mixture, roll out more pastry and make a lid for the pie. Press together round the edges, cut a few slits in the top, and bake for 25 - 30 minutes.

Barley Mushroom Bake

Low gluten

Ingredients:

1 large onion, finely chopped

2 tbs olive oil

1 carrot, grated

8 oz / 225g mushrooms, sliced

6 oz / 175g pot barley, washed and drained

8 fl oz/ 250ml vegetable stock

½ tsp dried marjoram

Sea salt to taste & black pepper

Method:

1. Gently fry the onion in the oil until it turns clear. Add the carrot and mushrooms. Continue cooking for 3 - 4 minutes or until the vegetables begin to soften.

2. Add the barley and stir to make sure it is well coated with oil. Transfer the mixture to a casserole dish and pour on the stock. Add the herbs, salt and pepper. Stir and cover. Bake at 350°F/180°C for 1 hour or until the barley is tender.

Vegetarian Nut Roast

Ingredients:

1 tbs olive oil

1 & 1/3 rd cups / 270g toasted hazelnuts, ground

2/3rd cup / 100g walnuts, ground

2/3rd cup / 100g brazil nuts, ground

12 oz / 350g tomatoes, blanched, peeled, and chopped

1 large onion, finely chopped

¼ lb / 110g fresh mushrooms, chopped

½ tsp dried basil

½ tsp dried oregano

1 tsp sea salt

egg substitute for 1 egg

clove garlic minced

Method:

Preheat oven to 425 F / 220c.

1. Lightly oil a 2 lb / 1 litre loaf tin or round mould. Line with waxed paper and set aside.

2. Place the nuts, tomatoes, onion, garlic, mushrooms, basil, oregano, sea salt, and egg substitute in a medium-sized bowl. Mix until the ingredients are thoroughly combined.

3. Turn the mixture into the prepared loaf tin, smoothing the surface with the back of a spoon. Place the tin in oven and bake for 30-40 minutes or until roast has shrunk slightly from the sides of the tin.

4. Let cool slightly and with a knife around the edges, turn out to a wooden board or plate. Cut into thick slices and serve with mushroom or onion gravy

Lentil-Nut Loaf

Ingredients:

2 cups / 400g red lentils, washed

4 cups / 1000ml water

2 large onions, chopped

2 cups / 200g mushrooms, chopped

4 tbs oil

Roughly 2 cups/ 250g nuts, ground - your choice

2 cups / 140g wheat-free breadcrumbs

2 tbs lemon juice

1 tbs tamari

sea salt and pepper to taste

2 tbs mixed herbs

Method:

Cook lentils in water until soft (½ hour). Sauté onions and mushrooms in oil until soft. Mix with remaining ingredients. Place in a greased baking pan and bake at 350F / 180c for 30 minutes. Garnish with parsley.

Chilled Vegetable Loaf

This is another version of the vegetarian loaf - this one involves no cooking - it is eaten raw which will provide better nutritional value and extra fibre

Ingredients:

3 - 4 carrots, roughly chopped

1-2 sweet potatoes, grated

1-2 white potatoes, grated

1 turnip, grated

1 onion, cut-up

3 celery stalks, with leaves

1 lb/ 450g raw peanuts

Sea salt to taste

Freshly ground black pepper to taste

Method:

Put each item in a food processor individually. When each item is processed, place in a large bowl. Mix together and refrigerate overnight. Next day, shape into a loaf. This recipe can be adapted to suit your taste. You can add herbs and/or spices

Triple Grain and Mushroom Pilaff

Very low in gluten

This is a recipe compiled to provide a dish for catering as it is a very tasty and provides 8 - 10 servings. Simply reduce the amount of ingredients to make a smaller batch.

Ingredients:

6 cups / 1500ml vegetable stock, divided

1 cup / 200g pearl barley, rinsed and drained

¾ cup / 160g millet, rinsed and drained

¾ cup / 160g quinoa, rinsed and drained

1 tsp salt

1 ½ cups / 150g green onions, thinly sliced

2 tbs olive oil

12 oz. / 350g mushrooms, washed and sliced

1 ½ tbs garlic, minced

2 tbs sesame seeds

2 tbs toasted sesame oil

6 cups / 500g spinach, well washed, and roughly chopped

1/3rd cup / 80ml freshly chopped parsley

2 tbs freshly chopped thyme

2 tbs tamari

½ tsp freshly ground black pepper

1/8th tsp cayenne pepper

Method:

1. In a saucepan, place 3 cups vegetable stock and pearl barley, and bring to a boil. Reduce heat to low, cover, and simmer for 45-50 minutes or until barley is tender. Remove from heat, drain off any excess water, and set aside.

2. Meanwhile, in another saucepan, place the remaining vegetable stock, millet, quinoa, and salt, and bring to a boil. Reduce heat to low, cover, and simmer for 15 minutes or until the grains are tender and most of the liquid has been absorbed. Drain off any excess water, leave the grains in the saucepan covered, and let sit for 5 minutes to allow the grains to steam.

3. In a large non-stick skillet, gently cook the green onions and onion in olive oil for 5 minutes to soften. Add the mushrooms and sauté an additional 3 minutes. Add the garlic and sesame seeds, and sauté an additional 2-3 minutes or until the vegetables are tender. Add the toasted sesame oil and all three cooked grains to the skillet, and sauté for 3 minutes to heat through.

4. Add the remaining ingredients and continue to cook until the spinach wilts. Taste and adjust the seasonings, as needed. Transfer the pilaf to a large bowl for service.

Orange and Almond Barley Pilaff

Very low in gluten

Ingredients:

1 oz / 25g blanched almonds, halved

5 cardamon pods

4 oz /110g pot barley, washed and drained

1 pint vegetable stock

½ tsp ground turmeric

Pinch ground ginger

Juice of 1 orange

Grated zest of 1 orange

Sea salt to taste

Freshly ground black pepper to taste

Method:

1. Heat a frying pan over a moderate heat and dry fry the almonds for 5 minutes, shaking the pan frequently. Set them aside.

2. Split the cardamon pods and release the seeds. Toast the seeds in the frying pan over a moderate heat for about 5 minutes, stirring frequently. Remove the seeds and crush them in a grinder or pestle and mortar.

3. Put the pearl barley into the frying pan with the crushed cardamom seeds, the stock, turmeric, ginger, orange rind and juice. Season to taste with salt and pepper. Bring to the boil, stir well and cover. Simmer over a low heat for about 1 ½ hours or until the barley is tender and the stock has been absorbed.

4. If there is any remaining liquid, turn up the heat and boil it off. Turn onto a heated dish and scatter with the toasted almonds.

Spicy Nut Pilaff

Gluten free

Serves 6

Ingredients:

½ cup/ 60g pistachios, roughly chopped

½ cup / 60g sliced almonds

¼ cup / 30g sunflower seeds

1 cup / 100g spring onions, sliced

1 cup / 100g carrot, shredded

2/3rds cup celery, finely diced

2 tbs olive oil

1 tbs garlic, minced

1 ½ tsp ground cumin

1 tsp ground coriander

½ tsp ground cardamom

2 cups / 450g basmati rice, rinsed

2 ½ / 650ml cups vegetable stock

¼ cup / 70ml tamari

½ tsp sea salt

¼ tsp pepper

1/3rd cup / 40g freshly chopped coriander

¼ cup / 30g freshly chopped parsley

Method:

1. In large pan, place the pistachios, almonds, and sunflower seeds, and cook over low heat for 3-4 minutes or until fragrant and lightly toasted. Transfer the nuts to a bowl and set aside.

2. In the same saucepan gently cook the spring onion, carrot, and celery in the olive oil for 3 minutes or until softened. Add the garlic, cumin, coriander, and cardamom, and cook an additional 1-2 minutes or until fragrant.

3. Add the basmati rice, stir well to thoroughly combine, and cook an additional 2 minutes while stirring constantly. Add the vegetable stock, tamari, salt, and pepper, and bring to a boil. Cover, reduce the heat to low, and simmer for 10 minutes.

4. Remove from the heat and set aside to steam for 5 minutes. After 5 minutes, remove the lid, fluff the rice with a fork, and stir in the reserved nuts, coriander, and parsley. Transfer to a large bowl or platter for service.

Fruit and Nut Pilaff

Gluten free

This is a special dish that is very suited to special occasions

Serves 6

Ingredients:

2 ½ cups / 500g millet

½ cup/ 40g sliced almonds

1 cup / 100g onion, finely diced

1 cups / 100g shallots, finely diced

2 tbs olive oil

2 cups / 200g apples, peeled, cored, and diced

2 tbs ginger, minced

1 tbs garlic, minced

1 bay leaf

1 cinnamon stick

4 cups / 1000ml vegetable stock or water

1 cup / 250ml apple juice

½ tsp sea salt

¼ tsp pepper

¼ cup / 40g raisins

¼ cup / 30g freshly chopped parsley

Method:

1. In a non-stick saucepan, place the millet, and cook over medium heat for 3-4 minutes or until fragrant. Remove the millet from the pan and set aside. In the same saucepan, place the almonds, and cook over medium heat for 3-4 minutes or until lightly toasted and fragrant. Remove the almonds from the pan and set aside.

2. Return the saucepan to the heat and cook the onion and shallots in olive oil for 5 minutes or until soft. Add the apple, ginger, garlic, bay leaf, and cinnamon stick, and cook an additional 3 minutes. Add the reserved millet, vegetable stock, apple juice, salt, and pepper to the saucepan, and bring to a boil. Cover, reduce heat to low, and simmer for 15-20 minutes or until all of the liquid is absorbed.

3. Remove the pan from the heat and set aside for 10 minutes to allow the millet to steam. Remove the bay leaf and cinnamon stick and discard. Fluff the pilaf with a fork, add the remaining ingredients, the reserved toasted almonds, and fluff the pilaf again to incorporate them. Taste and adjust seasonings if necessary

Vegetable and Nut Couscous – not using wheat based couscous

Gluten free

Today much of the couscous available is produced from durum flour which contains less gluten than wheat flour. Originally couscous was made from millet. In some regions of the world couscous is also made from coarsely ground barley, pearl millet or from rice flour.

You can now buy *Gluten free* couscous from various sources – your local health store or from *Gluten free* food retailers online. Also, the soaking process of preparing couscous helps to reduce the level of phytic acid that may be found in the dried product.

Serves 4

Ingredients:

1 cup / 150g onion, diced

1 tbs olive oil

4 cups / 700g broccoli, chopped

1½ cups/ 250g red pepper, (bell) chopped

1 tbs garlic, minced

2 cups / 500ml water or vegetable stock

3 tbs lemon juice

1 tsp sea salt

½ tsp freshly ground black pepper

1½ cups/200g couscous – Gluten free

¾ cup / 60g almonds, roughly chopped

¼ cup / 30g freshly chopped dill

¼ cup / 30g freshly chopped parsley

Method:

1. In a large saucepan, gently cook the onion in the olive oil for 3 minutes to soften. Add the broccoli stems and continue to cook the mixture an additional 3 minutes. Add the broccoli florets, red pepper, and garlic, and continue to cook an additional 4 minutes while stirring often.

2. Add the water, lemon juice, salt, and pepper, and bring the mixture to a boil. Add the couscous, stir, cover, remove the saucepan from the heat, and set aside for 5 minutes. Using a fork, fluff the couscous while stirring in the remaining ingredients. Taste and adjust seasonings, to taste. Serve hot, cold, or at room temperature as a side dish or with salad.

The Spicy Selection

I have included a good selection of Asian main meal recipes here to spice up your diet, especially as many spices have medicinal properties.

Chillies - Chillies are a great addition to a health enhancing diet - even in the smallest doses. One chilli has 100 % of the daily recommended dose of the anti-oxidant beta-carotene plus as much as 200 % of the required daily dose of vitamin C.

Chillies contain a plant chemical called capsaicin, which according to recent research has the ability to **temporarily block chemically transmitted pain signals** in the body. This is why you will find it in natural ointments to relieve arthritis and nerve pain.

Interestingly, there is good evidence that capsaicin may even soothe pains of the mind and soul since it appears to trigger the release of the mood-enhancing endorphins in the brain. Is this why some people get almost addicted to curries!

Garlic - Garlic has been prescribed for thousands of years as a cure for just about everything. Garlic has much more powerful antibiotic properties when you eat it raw than when you cook it.

Garlic lowers total cholesterol while increasing HDL (the 'good' cholesterol), it lowers blood pressure, inhibits the growth of cancer cells within the body and stimulates the immune system.

Fenugreek - Fenugreek is rich in diosgenin, a phytochemical from which chemists in the laboratory derive nature-identical progesterone - interesting!

Fenugreek also enhances digestion and is one of the best deep cleansers for the body that you can find in nature. So consider adding some to your spice cooking. You can make fenugreek tea using the seeds.

Ginger - Ginger is brilliant at alleviating the symptoms of colds and flu, it increases circulation and calms fevers. It relieves indigestion and flatulence, stimulates the circulation and is used in natural medicine to counter rheumatism. Many scientists studying this amazing root believe that ginger works its wonders due to an ability to block inflammatory tendencies in the body. This benefit should be utilised for women with endometriosis, to help with the inflammatory action of the disease.

The use of oils in Asian Cooking

Indian cooks use a variety of oils in their cooking. You can use the oils which are beneficial in a diet for Endometriosis, using oils which incorporate omega-3 acids. These include Safflower oil, Walnut oil, and Flax seed oil.

Indian cooking uses, among others, Mustard oil, Sesame oil and Coconut oil. I highly recommend the use of Coconut oil for its health benefits, and many people with Candida are using this oil with good results.

Clinical studies have shown that Coconut oil has anti-microbial and anti-viral properties, and is now even being used in treating AIDS patients. Studies conducted in the Philippines showed that coconut oil does indeed reduce the viral load in AIDS patients.

Lauric Acid a Key Component to Health

Lauric acid is a medium chain fatty acid which is abundant in coconut oil, and considered to be responsible for many of its health benefits. Coconut oil is about 50% lauric acid. The only other abundant source found in nature is in human breast milk.

The final choice of which oil you use will also depend on your budget as well as your preference for taste.

Indian Dishes

Yellow Split Pea Casserole

Ingredients:

2 tbs oil

1 tbs black mustard seeds

1 onion finely chopped

2 garlic cloves crushed

1 carrot grated

1 inch piece of ginger root grated

1 green chilli, de-seeded and chopped finely

1 tbs tomato puree

1 cup / 250g yellow split peas – soaked in water for 2 hours

13oz / 375g can chopped tomatoes

2 cups /500ml vegetable stock

1½ cups / 200g pumpkin cubed

225g cauliflower, cut into florets

1 large aubergine, cubed

1 tbs fresh chopped coriander

1 tbs garam masala

Salt and pepper

Method:

1. Heat the oil in a large pan. Add the mustard seeds, and when they start to splutter, add the onion, garlic, carrot and ginger. Cook until soft, about 5 mins. Add the green chilli and stir in the tomato puree. Stir in the split peas.

2. Add the tomatoes and stock, and bring to the boil. Season well.

3. Simmer for 40 mins, stirring occasionally. Add the pumpkin cubes and cauliflower florets, and simmer for a further 30 mins, covered, until the split peas are soft

4. Meanwhile, heat the oil in a frying pan over a high heat. Add the aubergine, and stir until sealed on all sides; remove and drain on paper towels.

5. Stir the aubergine into the split pea mixture with the coriander and garam masala. Check for seasoning.

6. Transfer to a serving dish and serve immediately.

Cauliflower with Indian Spices

Ingredients:

1 tbs oil

1 tsp ground cumin

½ tsp ground coriander

½ tsp ground ginger

1 small tomato, finely chopped

1 medium head cauliflower, separated into small florets

Salt and pepper

Method:

1. In a large skillet or wok, melt butter and oil over medium heat. Add cumin, coriander, and ginger. Cook spices until fragrant, about one minute.

2. Add tomato and cauliflower florets to skillet. Gently mix until cauliflower is evenly coated with spice mixture. Add ¼ cup / 70ml water. Cover; cook 20 minutes, until cauliflower is tender. Season to taste with salt and pepper

Roasted Aubergine Curry

Ingredients:

2 whole aubergines

1 cup / 250ml yoghurt substitute

(see Alternative Ingredients)

2 cardamon pods

½ tsp ground turmeric

1 dried red chilli

½ tsp coriander seeds

½ tsp pepper

1 tsp garam masala

1 clove

2 tbs oil

1 onion, sliced lengthways

2 garlic cloves, crushed

1 tbs grated ginger root

6 ripe tomatoes, peeled, de-seeded and quartered

Sprigs of fresh coriander to garnish

Method:

1. If you have a gas cooker, roast the 2 aubergines over a naked flame, turning frequently, until charred and black all over. Alternatively, cook in a very hot oven for 15 mins, turning once. Then peel under running cold water. Cut off the stem and discard.

2. Put the peeled aubergines into a large bowl and mash lightly with a fork. Stir in the yoghurt. Set aside

3. Grind together the cardamom pods, turmeric, red chilli, coriander seeds, pepper, garam masala and clove in a large pestle and mortar or spice grinder

4. Heat the oil in a wok or heavy frying pan over a moderate heat and cook the onion, garlic and ginger root until soft. Add the tomatoes and ground spices, and stir well

5. Add the aubergine mixture to the pan and stir well. Cook for 5 mins over a gentle heat, stirring constantly, until all the flavours are combined, and some of the liquid has evaporated. Serve immediately garnished with coriander

Curried Chickpeas and Carrots with Almonds

This is really a spicy salad dish but I have added it here as I think it would go well with other hot spicy vegetable dishes, but it is a meal in itself.

Ingredients:

½ cup / 65g sprouted chickpeas -(see Sprouting in Tips and Techniques)

2 large carrots, thinly sliced

1 red bell pepper, diced

3 spring onions, finely chopped

¼ cup / 30g sprouted almonds, blanched

½ cup / 30g nut yoghurt

½ cup/ 150ml orange juice

1 tbsp. olive oil & flaxseed oil mixed together

4 garlic cloves, minced

½ tsp. fresh ginger, minced

½ tsp. ground brown mustard seeds

½ tsp. ground cumin

½ tsp. ground coriander

½ tsp. turmeric cayenne pepper to taste

 Sea salt, to taste

Method:

1. Put the chick-peas into a food processor and chop. Not too much - you just want to gently break apart the peas so that they are easier to chew.

2. Slice the carrots very thin. Chop almonds into match-stick size pieces.

3. Put the chick-peas, carrots, bell pepper, spring onions and almonds into a large glass bowl and blend in 1/2 cup of yoghurt. Set aside.

4. In a separate bowl, stir the orange juice with the oil and spices. Add this into the chick-pea and vegetable mixture and mix well. Serves 3-4. Keeps for 2-3 days in the refrigerator.

Coconut Rice

Ingredients:

8oz / 225g basmati rice

3 tbs oil

1 onion, chopped

2 garlic cloves, crushed

1 inch piece ginger root, chopped

½ cinnamon stick

2 carrots grated

1 pint / 600ml boiling water or veg stock

1 oz / 25g creamed (block) coconut, chopped finely

Finely grated rind of ½ lemon or lime

1 tbs chopped fresh coriander

1 bunch spring onions, sliced

Method:

1. Place the rice in a sieve and wash well under cold running water until water runs clear. Drain well

2. Heat the oil in a large saucepan, add the onion, garlic, ginger and cinnamon and fry gently for 1 minute. Stir in the rice and carrots and mix until well coated with the oil.

3. Stir in the water or stock and season with salt and pepper. Bring to the boil, cover, reduce heat and simmer gently for 15 mins. without taking off the lid

4. Add the creamed coconut, lemon rind, chopped spring onions, fork through and serve immediately

Indian Dhal Dishes

There are various dhal (lentils and dried pulses) recipes from India. In the absence of regular supplies of meat, they form a staple part of the Indian diet. Lentils are full of protein, are easy to store and very versatile.

You can vary the types of dhal for each recipe. The soaking and cooking times do vary, so check the pack for instructions.

For those of you who cannot cope with food that is too spicy, then simply reduce the amount of spices, but most of these dishes are quite mild in flavour. Dhal is lovely served with a swirl of creamy Greek yoghurt as a treat! – see introduction about yoghurt.

Dhal with Spinach

Ingredients:

1 cup / 130g continental lentils

5 cups / 1250ml water

6 tbs oil

1 large onion, chopped

1 leek, shredded

12oz / 350g spinach, shredded coarsely

1 red (bell) pepper, chopped

2-3 garlic cloves, peeled and crushed

2 small chillies finely chopped

2 tsp cumin seeds

2 tsp ground coriander

Salt and pepper

Method:

1. Place the lentils in a sieve and rinse well under cold running water. Drain, then place in a saucepan with the water. Bring to the boil, cover and cook for 30 mins until the lentils are tender and the liquid has been absorbed

2. Meanwhile, heat some oil in a large saucepan and add the chopped onion, leek, shredded spinach and red (bell) pepper. Fry gently for about 8 mins, stirring and turning frequently until the spinach has wilted. Stir in the garlic, chilli and spices and fry gently for a further 2 mins

3. When the lentils are cooked, uncover and shake the pan over a moderate heat for a few moments to dry off. Add the lentils to the saucepan containing the spinach and onion mixture and toss together. Season with salt and pepper to taste and serve with mango chutney.

Tarka Dhal

Serves 4

Ingredients:

2 tbs oil

2 shallots, sliced

1 tsp yellow mustard seeds

2 garlic cloves, crushed

8 fenugreek seeds

½ inch piece ginger root, grated

½ tsp salt

½ cup / 65g red lentils (washed)

1 tbs tomato puree

1 pint / 600ml water

2 tomatoes, peeled and chopped

1 tbs lemon juice

4 tbs chopped fresh coriander

½ tsp chilli powder

½ tsp garam masala

Method:

1. Heat half the oil in a large saucepan, and add the shallots. Cook for 2-3 mins over a high heat, then add the mustard seeds. Cover the pan until the seeds begin to pop.
2. Immediately remove the lid from the pan and add the garlic, fenugreek, ginger and salt.
3. Stir once and add the lentils, tomato puree and water and simmer gently for 10 mins.
4. Stir in the tomatoes, lemon juice, and coriander and simmer for a further 4 to 5 mins until the lentils are tender.
5. Transfer to a serving dish. Heat the remaining oil in a small pan until it start to bubble. Remove from the heat and stir in the chilli powder and garam masala. (Leave this part out if you do not want the dish too spicy) Immediately pour over the dhal and serve with wheat-free India style bread like nan bread

Note - To make a dhal stew into a single dish meal, add a combination of vegetables such as steamed aubergine cubes, courgettes, carrots or any firm vegetable that you have to hand. Pumpkin is particularly successful.

Channa Dhal

Using Yellow split peas this time

Serves 4-6

Ingredients:

2 tbs oil

1 large onion, finely chopped

1 garlic clove, crushed

1 tbs grated ginger root

1 tbs cumin seeds, ground

1 dried red chilli, chopped

1 inch piece cinnamon stick

1 tsp salt

½ tsp ground turmeric

1 cup split yellow peas -

soaked in cold water for 1 hour and drained

14oz / 400g can tomatoes

1 & 1/3rd / 80ml cups water

2 tsp garam masala

Method:

1. Heat the oil in a large saucepan, add the onion, garlic and ginger and fry for 3-4 mins until the onion has softened slightly.
2. Add the cumin, coriander, chilli, cinnamon, salt and turmeric, then stir in the split peas until well mixed
3. Add the contents of the can of tomatoes, breaking the tomatoes up slightly with back of the spoon.
4. Add the water and bring to the boil. Reduce the heat to very low and simmer, uncovered, for about 40 mins, stirring occasionally, until most of the liquid has been absorbed and the split peas are tender. Skim the surface occasionally with a perforated spoon to remove any scum
5. Gradually stir in the garam masala, tasting after each addition, until it is of the required flavour

Note. If the dish is over-stirred during cooking the split peas will break up and the dish will not have much texture or bite

Spinach and Cauliflower Bhaji

Serves 4

Ingredients:

1 cauliflower

1 lb / 450g fresh spinach

4 tbs oil

2 large onions, chopped coarsely

2 garlic cloves, crushed

1 inch piece ginger root, chopped

1 tsp chilli powder, or to taste

1 tsp ground cumin

1 tsp ground turmeric

2 tsp ground coriander

14oz / 400g can chopped tomatoes

½ pint / 300ml veg stock

Salt and pepper

Method:

1. Divide the cauliflower into small florets, discard the hard central stalk. Trim the stalks from the spinach leaves. Heat the oil in a large saucepan, add the onions and cauliflower florets and fry the vegetables gently for about 3 mins, stirring frequently.
2. Add the garlic, ginger and spices and cook gently for 1 minute. Stir in the tomatoes and the stock and season with salt and pepper. Bring to the boil, cover, reduce the heat and simmer gently for about 10 mins.
3. Add the spinach to the pan, stirring and turning to wilt the leaves. Cover and simmer gently for about 10 mins, stirring frequently until the spinach has wilted and the cauliflower is tender. Serve hot.

Spicy Spinach and Aubergine

Serves 4

Ingredients:

1 cup / 130g split red lentils

3 cups / 750ml water

1 onion

1 aubergine

1 red pepper (bell)

2 courgettes

4 oz / 110g mushrooms

8oz / 220g spinach leaf

4 tbs oil

1 fresh green chilli, de-seeded and chopped

1 tsp ground cumin

1 tsp ground coriander

1 inch piece ginger root, chopped

2/3rds cup/ 170ml vegetable stock

Sea salt

Method:

1. Wash the lentils and place in a saucepan with water. Cover and simmer for 15 mins until the lentils are soft but still whole

2. Meanwhile, peel, quarter and slice the onion. Trim leaf end from the aubergine and cut into 1cm pieces. Remove stalk end and seeds from the bell pepper and cut into ½ inch pieces. Trim and cut courgettes into ½ inch slices. Thickly slice the mushrooms. Discard course stalks from spinach leaves and wash spinach well

3. Heat the oil in a large saucepan; add the onion and red (bell) pepper and fry gently for 3 mins, stirring frequently. Stir in the aubergine, courgettes, mushrooms, chilli, spices and ginger and fry gently for 1 minute. Add the spinach and stock and season with salt to taste

4. Stir and turn until the spinach leaves wilt down. Cover and simmer for 10 mins or until the vegetables are just tender. Make a border of the lentils on a warm serving plate and spoon the vegetable mixture into the centre. (The lentils may be stirred into the vegetable mixture, instead of being used as a border, if wished)

Spiced Chickpeas

Chickpeas are very versatile and I use them in many vegetable based casseroles to add protein, fibre and bulk. Here is a tasty Indian variation.

I am inclined to advise buying tinned, ready cooked chickpeas as they can take ages to cook. It is better to cook your own beans and pulses as much as possible, but the cost of cooking them could add up on your power bills. (Tips on bulk cooking beans near back of the book)

For this recipe you can also use black-eye beans which have a smoother, creamier flavour. Omit the chillies for a less fiery flavour.

Serves 4

Ingredients:

1 large aubergine

2 courgettes

6 tbs oil

1 large onion, quartered and sliced

2 garlic cloves, crushed

1 - 2 fresh chillies, de-seeded and chopped

2 tsp ground coriander

2 tsp cumin seeds

1 tsp ground turmeric

1 tsp garam masala

14oz / 400g can chopped tomatoes

1¼ cups / 300ml vegetable stock

14 oz / 400g can chick peas, drained and rinsed

2 tbs chopped fresh mint

¼ pint / 150ml yoghurt or yoghurt substitute

Salt and pepper

Method:

1. Trim the leaf end off aubergine and cut into cubes. Trim and slice the courgettes. Heat the oil in a saucepan and gently fry the aubergine, courgettes, onion, garlic and chillies for about 5 mins, stirring frequently and adding a little more oil if necessary.

2. Stir in the spices and cook for 30 seconds. Add the tomatoes, stock and salt and pepper to taste and cook for 10 mins.

3. Add the chick peas to the pan and continue cooking for a further 5 mins. Stir in the mint and yoghurt and reheat gently. Taste and adjust the seasoning. Serve hot with plain or pilau rice.

Note. When using yoghurt in cooking, blend ½ teaspoon of cornflour to yoghurt before adding to pan and heat gently, stirring constantly. The corn flour helps stabilise the yoghurt to prevent it separating during heating.

You can also add some ground almonds to this and other Indian dishes, which adds to the richness and flavour, as well as added goodness

Vegetable, Nut & Lentil Koftas

Serves 4-5

The mixture here is shaped into golf-ball shapes and baked in the oven with a sprinkling of aromatic garam masala. They are delicious served hot or cold with a yoghurt dressing and chapattis. You can make these Koftas and freeze some for another day.

Ingredients:

6 tbs oil

1 onion, chopped finely

2 carrots, chopped finely

2 celery sticks, chopped finely

2 garlic cloves, crushed

1 fresh green chilli, de-seeded and chopped

1½ tbs curry powder or paste

1¼ cups / 160g split red lentils

2 ½ cups / 640ml vegetable stock

2 tbs tomato puree

2 cups / 500ml fresh bread-crumbs (from non-wheat bread)

¾ cup / 90g unsalted cashews, chopped

2 tbs chopped fresh coriander

1 egg beaten or egg substitute

Salt and pepper

Garam masala for sprinkling

Yoghurt dressing:
Ingredients:

8oz / 225g natural yoghurt or yoghurt substitute

1-2 tbs chopped fresh coriander

1-2 tbs mango chutney, chopped if necessary

Method:

1. Heat 4 tablespoons of oil in a large saucepan and gently fry the onion, carrots, celery, garlic and chilli for 5 mins, stirring frequently. Add the curry powder or paste and the lentils and cook gently for 1 minute, stirring.

2. Add the stock and tomato paste and bring to the boil. Reduce the heat, cover and simmer for 20 mins or until the lentils are tender and all the liquid is absorbed.

3. Remove from the heat and cool slightly. Add the breadcrumbs, nuts, coriander, egg and seasoning to taste. Mix well and leave to cool. Using 2 spoons, shape into rounds about the size of a golf ball.

4. Place the balls on a greased baking sheet, drizzle with the remaining oil and sprinkle with a little garam masala, to taste. Cook in a preheated oven at 350°F/180°C. for 15 to 20 mins or until piping hot and lightly golden.

5. Meanwhile, make the yoghurt dressing. Mix all the ingredients together in a bowl. Garnish with coriander sprigs. Serve the koftas hot with the yoghurt dressing

Jacket Potatoes with Beans

Baked jacket potatoes, topped with a tasty mixture of beans in a spicy sauce, provide a deliciously filling, high fibre dish.

Serves 6

Ingredients:

6 large potatoes (for baking)

4 tbs oil

1 large onion, chopped

2 garlic cloves, crushed

1 tsp turmeric

1tbs cumin seeds

2 tbs mild curry paste

12oz / 350g cherry tomatoes

14oz / 400g can black-eye beans, drained and rinsed

14oz / 400g can red kidney beans, drained and rinsed

1 tbs lemon juice

2 tbs tomato puree

¼ pint/ 150ml water

2 tbs fresh chopped coriander

Salt and pepper

Method:

1. Wash and scrub the potatoes and prick several times with a fork. Cook in a preheated oven at 400°F/200°C for about 1 to 1 ¼ hours or until potatoes feel soft.

2. About 20 minutes before the end of cooking time, prepare the topping. Heat the oil in a saucepan, add the onion and cook gently for about 5 mins, stirring frequently. Add the garlic, turmeric, cumin seeds and curry paste and cook gently for 1 minute. Stir in the tomatoes, black-eye beans and red kidney beans, lemon juice, tomato puree, water and chopped coriander. Season with salt and pepper, then cover and cook gently for 10 mins, stirring frequently.

3. When the potatoes are cooked, cut a cross in the top and squeeze gently to open out. Mash the flesh slightly with a fork. Spoon the prepared bean mixture on top, serve at once. Try adding a green salad and a yoghurt dressing spooned over the potatoes.

Lentil & Vegetable Biryani

A delicious mix of vegetables, basmati rice and continental lentils produced a wholesome and nutritious dish

Serves 6 – ideal for catering

Ingredients:

2/3rds cup / 85g continental lentils

4 tbs oil

2 onions, quartered and sliced

2 garlic cloves, crushed

1 inch piece of ginger root, chopped

1 tsp ground turmeric

½ tsp chilli powder

1 tsp ground coriander

2 tsp ground cumin

3 tomatoes, skinned and chopped

1 aubergine, trimmed and cut into 1 cm pieces

2 ½ pints / 1400ml boiling vegetable stock

1 red (bell) pepper, diced

1 & ¾ cups / 220g basmati rice

1 cup / 150g green beans, halved

1 ½ cups / 325g cauliflower florets

4oz / 110g mushrooms, wiped and sliced

2oz / 50g unsalted cashew nuts

Sprigs of fresh coriander to garnish

Method:

1. Rinse the lentils under cold running water and drain. Heat the oil in saucepan, add the onions and fry gently for 2 mins. Stir in the garlic, ginger and spices and fry gently for 1 minute, stirring frequently. Add the lentils, tomatoes, aubergine and 2 ½ cups / 640ml of the stock, mix well, then cover and simmer gently for 20 mins. Add the red pepper and cook for a further 10 mins or until the lentils are tender and all the liquid has been absorbed

2. Meanwhile, place the rice in a sieve and rinse under cold running water until the water runs clear. Drain and place in another pan with the remaining stock. Bring to the boil, add the green beans, cauliflower and mushrooms, then cover and cook gently for 15 mins or until the

rice and vegetables are tender. Remove for the heat and leave, covered, for 10 mins.

3. Add the lentil mixture and the cashews to the cooked rice and mix lightly together. Pile onto a warm serving platter and garnish with coriander

Stuffed Aubergines

Serves 6 – ideal for catering

Ingredients:

1 & 1/3rd cups / 130gm continental lentils

1½ pints / 750ml water

2 garlic cloves, crushed

3 well-shaped aubergines

¼ pint / 140ml oil

2 onions, chopped

4 tomatoes, chopped

2 tsp cumin seeds

1 tsp ground cinnamon

2 tbs mild curry powder

1 tsp chilli - finely chopped

2 tbs chopped fresh mint

Salt and pepper

Method:

1. Rinse the lentils under cold running water. Drain and place in a saucepan with the water and garlic. Cover and simmer for 30 mins.

2. Cook the aubergines in a saucepan of boiling water for 5 mins. Drain, then plunge into cold water for 5 mins. Drain again. Cut in half lengthways. Scoop out most of the flesh and reserve, leave a 1cm thick border to form a shell.

3. Place the aubergine shells in a shallow greased ovenproof dish, brush with a little oil and sprinkle with salt and pepper. Cook in a pre-heated oven at 350°F/180°C for 10 mins. Meanwhile, heat half the remaining oil in a frying pan, add the onions and tomatoes and fry gently for 5 mins. Chop the reserved aubergine flesh, add to the pan with the spices and cook gently for 5 mins. Season with salt and pepper.

4. Stir in the lentils, most of the remaining oil, reserving a little for later, and the mint. Spoon the mixture into the shells. Drizzle with the remaining oil and bake for 15 mins. Serve hot or cold topped with a spoonful of natural yoghurt, sprinkled with chilli powder.

Brown Rice with Fruit and Nuts

Here is a tasty and filling rice dish that is nice and spicy. It includes fruits for a refreshing flavour and toasted nuts for an interesting crunchy texture

Serves 4-6

Ingredients:

4 tbs oil

1 large onion, chopped

2 cloves garlic, crushed

1 inch piece ginger root, chopped

1 tsp chilli powder

1 tsp cumin seeds

1 tbs mild curry paste

1 ½ cups / 330g brown rice

3 ½ cups / 900ml boiling vegetable stock

14oz / 400g can chopped tomatoes

6oz / 150g ready-soaked dried apricots

or peaches, cut into slivers

1 red (bell) pepper diced

3oz / 150g fresh peas

1-2 small, slightly green bananas

½ cup / 150ml toasted nuts

(a mixture of almonds, cashews and pine kernels)

Salt and pepper

Method:

1. Heat the oil in a large saucepan, add the onion and fry gently for 3 mins. Stir in the garlic, ginger, spices and rice and cook gently for 2 mins, stirring all the time until the rice is coated in the spiced oil.

2. Pour in the boiling stock and canned tomatoes and season with salt and pepper to taste. Bring to the boil, then reduce the heat, cover and simmer gently for 40 mins or until the rice is almost cooked and most of the liquid is absorbed.

3. Add the apricot or peach slivers, diced red pepper and peas. Cover and continue to cook for 10 mins. Remove for the heat and allow to stand for 5 mins without uncovering

4. Peel and slice the bananas. Uncover the rice mixture and fork through to mix the ingredients together. Add the toasted nuts and sliced banana and toss lightly. Transfer to a warm serving platter and garnish with coriander sprigs.

Okra with Green Mango and Lentils

This is a tangy and spicy dish which is a meal in itself. You can change the okra for a veg like courgette. Some people do not like okra – just experiment!

Serves 4

Ingredients:

4oz / 110g yellow lentils

3 tbs olive oil

½ tsp onion seeds

2 medium onions, sliced

½ tsp ground fenugreek

1 tsp ginger, finely chopped

1 tsp garlic, finely chopped

1 ½ tsp chilli powder

¼ tsp ground turmeric

1 tsp ground coriander

1 unripe mango, peeled and stoned then sliced

1 lb / 450g okra, chopped

2 fresh red chillies, seeded and sliced

2 tbs chopped fresh coriander

Method:

1. Wash the lentils and put into a saucepan with just enough water to cover. Bring to the boil and cook until soft but not mushy. Drain and set aside.

2. Heat oil in a preheated wok. Add the onion seeds and fry until they begin to pop. Add the onions and fry until they are golden brown. Lower the heat and add the ground fenugreek, ginger, garlic, chilli powder, turmeric and ground coriander. Keep stirring all the time.

3. Add the sliced mango and okra to the wok. Stir well. Then add the red chillies and fresh coriander. Stir fry for 3 minutes or until the okra is well cooked. Stir in the cooked lentils and cook for a further 3 minutes. Serve immediately.

Thai Dishes

Many Thai and Chinese recipes rely heavily on soy sauce, which is not suitable for an Endo diet, which I have explained earlier in the introduction. I have included here recipes which do not use soy and are very tasty and nutritious.

Notes:

Fish Sauce - this is a thin, strong flavoured salty sauce made from fermented anchovies. It is strong in flavour, so you can reduce the amounts below if you wish.

Coconut milk - this is not the same as the 'milk' from the inside of a fresh coconut. You can buy canned coconut milk or purchase coconut cream in a hard block and add warm water to it to turn it into milk.

Kaffir Lime Leaves - these are used rather like bay leaves, but give an aromatic lime flavour to dishes which is very distinctive. The fresh leaves are available from oriental food stores and can be frozen for future use. I have purchased some as dried whole leaves, and they work rather well.

Lemon Grass - This herb has a mild, sour-sweet, citrus flavour. It is what gives Thai cooking its distinct aroma and flavour in many dishes. It looks a little like a small spring-onion. Use only the lower 5 inches. Remove the stalks from the dish before serving as they are very woody.

Mixed Vegetables in Coconut Milk

A most delicious way of cooking vegetables. If you do not want your food so spiced, use fewer red chilli peppers.

Serves 4 - 6

Ingredients:

1lb / 450g mixed vegetables, such as aubergines,

 baby sweet-corn, carrots, squash, green beans, carrots

6 red chillies, seeded

2 stalks lemon grass, chopped

4 kaffir lime leaves, torn

2 tbs olive oil

1 cup / 250ml coconut milk

2 tbs fish sauce

Sea salt

Thai basil leaves, to garnish (optional)

Method:

1. Cut the vegetables into similar size shapes.

2. Put the red chillies, lemon grass and kaffir lime leaves in a mortar and grind together with a pestle.

3. Heat the oil in a wok or large deep frying pan. Add the chilli mixture and fry 2 - 3 minutes.

4. Stir in the coconut milk and bring to the boil. Add the vegetables and cook for about 5 minutes or until they are tender. Season with fish sauce and salt, and garnish with basil leaves.

5. *Add a flavoured rice dish and you have a complete meal.*

Spiced Cauliflower Braise

Serves 4

Ingredients:

1 cauliflower

2 medium tomatoes

1 onion, chopped

2 garlic cloves, crushed

1 fresh green chilli, seeded

½ tsp ground turmeric

2tbs olive oil

14fl oz / 500ml coconut milk

1 cup / 250ml water

1 tsp sugar substitute

Method:

1. Trim the stalk from the cauliflower and divide into small florets. Skin the tomatoes (if liked). Chop the flesh into 1 in pieces.

2. Grind the chopped onion, garlic, green chilli, ground turmeric together to a paste in a food processor or pestle and mortar. Heat the oil in a wok or large frying pan and fry the spice paste to bring out the flavours, without allowing it to brown.

3. Add the cauliflower florets and toss well to coat in the spices. Stir in the coconut milk, water, sugar substitute and salt to taste. Simmer for 5 minutes.

4. Add the tomatoes to the pan and cook for 2 - 3 minutes only. Taste and check the seasoning and serve.

Spiced Coconut Mushrooms

Here is a simple and delicious way to cook mushrooms. This dish is quite moist and creamy, so just add rice and you have a tasty meal which is quick to prepare.

Serves 4

Ingredients:

2 tbs groundnut oil

2 garlic cloves, finely chopped

2 fresh chillies, seeded and sliced into rings

3 spring onions, finely chopped

8oz/ 225g mushrooms, thickly sliced

2/3rds cup / 170ml coconut milk

2 tbs chopped fresh coriander

Sea salt

Fresh black pepper

Method:

1. Heat a wok until hot, add the oil and swirl around the wok. Add the garlic and chillies and stir fry for a few seconds.

2. Add the spring onions and stir fry for 2 -3 minutes until softened. Add the mushrooms and stir-fry for 3 minutes.

3. Pour in the coconut milk and bring to the boil. Boil rapidly over a high heat until the liquid has reduced to nearly half and coats the mushrooms well. Season to taste with salt and pepper.

4. Sprinkle over the chopped coriander and toss the mushrooms gently. Serve at once.

Nutty Rice and Mushroom Stir-fry

Serves 4 - 6

Ingredients:

12 oz / 350g long grain rice, preferably basmati

3 tbs olive oil

1 small onion, roughly chopped

8oz / 225g mushrooms, sliced

2 oz / 50g hazelnuts, roughly chopped

2 oz / 50g pecan nuts, roughly chopped

2 oz / 50g almonds, roughly chopped

4 tbs fresh parsley, chopped

Sea salt

Ground black pepper

Method:

1. Rinse the rice, then cook for 10 - 12 minutes in 1½ pints / 800mls salted water in a saucepan with a tight-filling lid. When cooked, refresh under cold water. Heat the wok, then add half the oil. Stir-fry the rice for 2 - 3 minutes. Remove and set aside.

2. Add remaining oil and stir-fry the onion for 2 minutes until softened but not coloured. Mix in the mushrooms and stir-fry for 2 minutes.

3. Add all the nuts and stir-fry for 1 minute. Return the rice to the wok and stir-fry for 3 minutes. Season with salt and pepper. Stir in the parsley and serve at once.

This is a simple dish that can be spiced up to your liking.

Stir-fried mixed Vegetables

Serves 4

Ingredients:

7oz / 200g broccoli

5oz / 150g french beans

7oz / 200g baby corn cobs

7oz / 200g pak choi

10oz / 275g baby carrots

3 spring onions

5 garlic cloves

5 tbs olive oil

3 tbs fish sauce

3 tbs oyster sauce

1 tbs sugar substitute - of choice

4 tbs chinese rice wine

Method:

1. Cut the broccoli into florets. Trim the beans and cut into quarters. Cut the baby corn in half crossways. Cut the pak choi into bite-size pieces. Cut the carrots lengthways into quarters. Cut the spring onions in half lengthways and then into pieces about 1 ¼ inches long.

2. Finely chop the garlic. Heat the oil in a large frying pan or wok over a high heat. Stir fry the garlic for 1 - 2 minutes, until golden brown. Add the broccoli, carrots, beans, and corn cobs and stir fry over a high heat for about 3 minutes. Stir in the spring onions, pak choi, fish sauce, oyster sauce and sugar substitute.

3. Add the rice wine and cook, stirring and tossing the vegetables constantly, for a further 2 minutes, until the vegetables are cooked but still crunchy.

Noodles with Courgettes

Gluten free using non-wheat based noodles like rice noodles. Not strictly Thai food, but it is cooked in a wok, is very quick to prepare and is full of flavour.

Serves 4

Ingredients:

2 yellow courgettes

2 green courgettes

4 tbs pine nuts

4 tbs olive oil

2 shallots, finely chopped

2 tbs capers, rinsed

2 garlic cloves, finely chopped

4 sun-dried tomatoes in oil, drained and cut into strips

12 oz / 350g wheat-free noodles

4 tbs chopped mixed herbs (such as tarragon, chives, thyme)

Grated rind of 1 lemon

Method:

1. Slice the courgettes diagonally into rounds the same thickness as the noodles. Then cut the courgette slices into match-sticks. Toast the pine nuts in an un-greased frying pan over a medium heat until golden in colour.

2. Heat half the oil in a wok. Add the shallots and garlic and fry until fragrant. Set aside. Add the remaining oil to the wok, and when hot, stir-fry the courgettes until soft.

3. Return the shallots to the wok and stir thoroughly. Add the caper, sun-dried tomatoes and pine nuts. Remove the pan from the heat.

4. Cook the noodles in a large saucepan in salted water until just tender. Drain well and toss into the courgette mixture, adding the herbs, lemon rind, with salt and pepper to taste. Serve at once.

Thai Stir-fry Curry

Most curries in Thailand include meat or seafood. I have adapted this recipe so that it is totally vegetarian. If you are including chicken in your diet, then you can include chicken (organic of course) in this recipe. Simply add 1 lb / 500g of chicken, chopped into smallish chunks, at stage 4 of this recipe, instead of the courgette.

Serves 4

Ingredients:

1 onion roughly cut.

1 & 2/3rds cups/ 170ml coconut milk

2 tbs red curry paste

2 tbs Thai fish sauce

1 tbs sweetener of choice

8 oz / 225g tiny new potatoes

12oz / 350g courgette, cut into ½ inch slices

1 tbs lime juice

2 tbs chopped fresh mint

1 tbs fresh basil

Sea salt

Ground black pepper

2 kaffir lime leaves, shredded

2 tbs olive oil

Method:

1. Heat the wok until hot, add the oil and swirl it around. Add the onion and stir-fry for 3 – 4 minutes.

2. Pour the coconut milk, then bring to the boil, stirring. Stir in the curry paste, fish sauce and sweetener.

3. Add the potatoes and seasoning and simmer for about 20 minutes.

4. Add the courgettes (or chicken), cover and cook over a low heat for a further 10 – 15 minutes, until vegetables are tender.

5. Stir in the lime juice, chopped mint and basil. Serve at once, sprinkled with the shredded kaffir lime leaves. Serve with rice.

Pasta Dishes

All these pasta dishes are gluten-free based on using wheat-free pasta

Many pasta dishes are quick and easy to prepare. Try experimenting by adding vegetables to the basic 'pasta' sauces. This will add extra nutritional value to the meal. I like to add steamed broccoli to many of my pasta dishes, and broccoli helps to modulate oestrogen levels in the body.

Don't forget to use wheat-free pasta. There are several varieties available in most health shops. Wheat-free pastas are made using various grains, such as rice, corn, quinoa, and spelt, and potatoes are also used.

Pasta with Lentil Sauce

4 servings

Ingredients:

1 tbs olive oil

1 onion chopped

1 clove garlic crushed

1 tbs basil

8oz / 225g chopped tomatoes

4 oz / 110g brown lentils

1 tbs tomatoes puree

20 fl oz / 560ml vegetable stock

Sea salt to taste

Freshly ground black pepper

Non wheat pasta of choice

Method:

1. Heat oil in pan and fry onion for 10 mins. Add garlic, basil, tomatoes, lentils, puree and stock. Bring to the boil, put on a lid, turn down heat and cook gently for 45 mins. Stir occasionally until lentils are tender and mixture is a thick puree.

2. Season with salt and pepper

3. Cook pasta, drain and serve with the sauce

Pasta with Sweet Peppers

4 servings

Ingredients:

1 tbs olive oil

Fresh coriander – small bunch chopped

2 bell peppers – 1 red, 1 yellow

¾ lb / 330g tomatoes – blended or tinned

Wheat-free pasta of choice

Method:

1. Clean and chop peppers and cook in pan with oil

2. Add tomatoes, salt and pepper and coriander

3. Cook pasta, drain, and add pepper mix, serve

You can add other herbs to this sauce for variations. Try basil or oregano.

Pasta with Sweet Pepper Blender Sauce

4 servings

Ingredients:

2 red (bell) peppers, chopped

6 tbs milk substitute

6 tomatoes

2 cloves garlic, chopped

Olive oil

Sea salt to taste

Freshly ground pepper to taste

Non wheat pasta of choice

Fresh coriander, chopped

Method:

1. Put all sauce ingredients, except the oil in a blender until it turns to a smooth paste. Continue to blend as you gradually incorporate a little oil at a time to make it the required thickness.

2. Transfer to pan and heat the sauce.

3. Cook and drain the pasta, serve with the sauce and sprinkle with chopped coriander

Pasta with Roasted Peppers and Coriander and Chilli Pesto

Serves 6

Ingredients:

3 mixed red and yellow (bell) peppers

2 oz / 50g trimmed fresh coriander, roughly chopped

1 fresh chilli, seeded and roughly chopped

2 garlic cloves, crushed

2 tbs pine nuts

Grated zest of 1 lime

1 tsp sea salt

8 tbs olive oil

Wheat-free spaghetti

Method:

1. Roast the peppers in a preheated oven at 425°F/225°C until the skins blackened on all sides.

2. Remove the skins and seeds, then chop the flesh into ½ inch dice

3. Put the coriander and chillies in a blender or food processor with the garlic, pine nuts, lime zest and salt. Puree until smooth, gradually adding the olive oil.

4. Cook and drain the spaghetti. Toss with the peppers and sauce and serve.

Spaghetti with Mustard Sauce

4 servings

Ingredients:

1½ lbs / 765g tomatoes - pureed in blender½ lb / 675g spring greens

6 tbs olive oil

1 red onion, finely chopped

3 garlic cloves, finely chopped

3 sage leaves, finely chopped

½ tsp dried chilli flakes

Sea salt to taste

Freshly ground black pepper

½ cup / 140ml yoghurt – see alternatives

Wheat-free pasta of choice

Method:

1. Plunge the broad beans into boiling water for 2 minutes. Drain under cold running water, then slip off the outer skins if they are tough.

2. Remove stalks from the greens and finely slice.

3. Heat oil in a large pan, and gently fry the onion until just soft. Add the garlic, sage and chilli flakes.

4. Add the greens and toss the leaves until coated with oil. Cover and cook over a medium heat for 7 - 10 minutes, until the greens are just tender, adding a little water if the mixture becomes too dry. Stir in the beans and season to taste. Add enough yoghurt to make the sauce a little creamy..

5. Cook the pasta, drain and toss with the vegetables.

Pasta with Courgette and Rosemary Sauce

Serves 4 - 6

Ingredients:

1 lb / 450g courgettes cut into matchstick strips

5 tbs olive oil

2 onions, very thinly sliced

1 clove garlic, finely chopped

1 tbs parsley, finely chopped

2 tbs fresh rosemary, finely chopped

Sea salt to taste

Freshly ground black pepper to taste

Wheat-free pasta of choice

Method:

1. Put the courgettes in a colander, sprinkle with salt and drain for 1 hour. Pat dry with paper towels.
2. In a pan, gently cook the onion with oil until golden. Add the garlic, parsley, courgettes, and fry until just tender, stirring frequently.
3. Stir in the rosemary and season to taste.
4. Cook the pasta and pour the sauce over the top and toss to mix in sauce.
5. Tip: add a little yoghurt to this sauce to make it more liquid at stage 3

Spaghetti with Peanut Sauce

Serves 5 - 6

Ingredients:

1 packet wheat free spaghetti

2 tsp. roasted peanut oil

1 cup / 120gg carrots grated

1 cup / 100g red bell peppers finely diced

¼ cup / 30g coriander chopped

¼ cup / 40g spring onions chopped

Sauce:

½ cup / 125g natural peanut butter

¼ cup/ 70ml tamari sauce

3 tbsp. fresh lime juice

2 tbsp. sweetener of choice

1-3 cloves garlic minced

Method:

1. Prepare pasta according to package directions. Drain and rinse with cold running water. Transfer to large bowl, drizzle with roasted peanut oil and toss to coat.
2. Make dressing using either a blender or a food processor. Combine peanut butter, tamari sauce, lime juice, sweetener and minced garlic. Blend until creamy.
3. Add carrots, peppers, cilantro, scallions and dressing to bowl of spaghetti and toss to coat. Garnish with chopped peanuts and lime wedges. Serve cold or at room temperature.

Pasta with Broad Beans and Greens

Serves 4

Ingredients:

8 oz / 225g shelled young broad beans

1 ½ lb / 675g spring greens

6 tbs olive oil

1 red onion, finely chopped

3 garlic cloves, finely chopped

3 sage leaves, finely chopped

½ tsp dried chilli flakes

Sea salt to taste

Freshly ground black pepper

½ cup yoghurt – see alternatives

Wheat-free pasta of choice

Method:

1. Plunge the broad beans into boiling water for 2 minutes. Drain under cold running water, then slip off the outer skins if they are tough.
2. Remove stalks from the greens and finely slice.
3. Heat oil in a large pan, and gently fry the onion until just soft. Add the garlic, sage and chilli flakes.
4. Add the greens and toss the leaves until coated with oil. Cover and cook over a medium heat for 7 - 10 minutes, until the greens are just tender, adding a little water if the mixture becomes too dry. Stir in the beans and season to taste. Add enough yoghurt to make the sauce a little creamy..
5. Cook the pasta, drain and toss with the vegetables.

Pasta with Grilled Vegetables and Herb Bread Crumbs

Serves 6.

This would be good for catering/entertaining

Ingredients:

1 lb / 450g of wheat-free pasta -uncooked

5 slices bread (wheat-free)

1 medium yellow squash, cut into 3/8 inch thick slices

1 medium courgette, cut ½ inch slices

1 small aubergine, cut ½ inch slices

1 medium onion, cut ½ inch slices

3 large red tomatoes, cut into ½ inch slices

½ bunch fresh basil, finely chopped, or 1 tsp dry basil

1 tbs fresh thyme, finely chopped, or 1 tsp dry thyme

1 tbs fresh oregano, finely chopped, or 1 tsp dry oregano

Sea salt and freshly ground black pepper to taste

2 tbs olive oil

4 tbs lemon juice

3 tbs balsamic vinegar

Method:

Preheat oven to 250°F/120°C

1. Cook pasta according to package directions; drain.

2. Tear bread slices into small pieces, place on baking sheet and bake until dry, about 20 minutes.

3. Meanwhile, brush courgette and yellow squash with a little vegetable oil and grill on both sides along with aubergine, onion and tomato slices. Do not over grill; keep fairly firm. Cool slightly and chop into 3/8 inch pieces.

4. When bread is dry, crumble it with your hands or chop in food processor until crumbled.

5. In a small bowl, combine basil, thyme and oregano, and salt and pepper to taste. Toss crumbs in basil mixture to coat. Heat oil in large pan. Add lemon juice, balsamic vinegar and grilled vegetables. Heat thoroughly. Adjust seasonings with salt and pepper, if desired.

6. Toss vegetables with cooked pasta. Divide into appropriate portion sizes. Top with seasoned bread crumbs. Serve immediately.

Lemon Pasta

Serves 4

Ingredients:

1 lb / 450g wheat-free pasta/spaghetti

1 cup / 25g fresh chopped parsley

2 medium cloves of garlic, minced

½ cup / 140ml olive oil

Zest & juice of two lemons

¾ cup / 75g toasted pine nuts

Salt & pepper

Garnish: lemon wedges

Method:

1. Mix together the oil, garlic, parsley and lemon zest and juice. Season with salt and pepper. Add the toasted pine nuts, stir well, and allow to sit for a couple of hours for the flavours to meld.

2. Cook the pasta in boiling salted water until it is al dente. Just before draining, remove a small cup of pasta water. Drain the pasta, and return it to the pot with the lemon sauce over high heat. Add a little pasta water to prevent it from drying out. As soon as it is piping hot, remove from the heat and serve with a wedge of lemon.

Fresh Herb and Lemon Sauce

This is a very quick recipe. You could serve this with some steamed broccoli or other vegetables to add fibre and extra nutrition

Serves 4 - 6

Ingredients:

8 spring onions, green parts included, finely chopped

Finely grated zest of 1 lemon

3 oz/ 75g trimmed mixed herbs (parsley, rocket, thyme, marjoram, basil) chopped

4 tbs toasted bread-crumbs (wheat-free)

Sea salt to taste

Freshly ground black pepper to taste

Wheat-free pasta of choice

½ cup / 150ml yoghurt – home-made or live yoghurt

2 tbs olive oil

Method:

1. Cook and drain the pasta and transfer to a heated serving dish.

2. Heat the oil until hot. Remove from the heat and immediately stir in the spring onions, lemon zest and herbs. Then add the yoghurt.

3. Toss with pasta and breadcrumbs and serve immediately.

Lemon Pasta with Grilled Vegetables

Serves 4

Ingredients:

1 box/packet pasta of choice

1 zucchini (courgette)

15 cherry tomatoes

1 to 2 green peppers – to taste

1 large onion

5 cloves garlic

1 lemon

1-2 tsp. lemon peel

Olive oil

Method:

1. Chop the courgette/zucchini, onion, and green peppers into chunks and toss them in olive oil with the cherry tomatoes. Stick all the vegetables on skewers and place under a grill until partially cooked (about 10 minutes).

2. Chop the garlic cloves finely and sauté in oil. Grate the peel of the lemon until you have 1-2 teaspoons of lemon rind, then juice the lemon. Cook pasta. When the pasta is done, toss it in about 1 tbsp. of olive oil. Then add the lemon juice, lemon rind, garlic, and grilled vegetables and toss.

Pasta with Leek and Parsley Sauce

Serves 4

Ingredients:

3 tbs olive oil

1 lb / 450gm leeks, sliced lengthways and cut into match-sticks

3 tbs fresh parsley

2 tsp green peppercorns, crushed

1 cup / 250ml yoghurt – home-made or live yoghurt

Sea salt to taste

Wheat-free pasta of choice.

Method:

1. Heat the oil in a pan and gently fry the leeks with the green peppercorns for 3 - 4 minutes until the leeks are just tender. Stir in the parsley and yoghurt and season to taste.

2. Cook the pasta, drain and toss with the sauce.

Tomato and Fennel Pasta

Serves 4 - Fresh fennel adds an intriguing, flavour to this sun-dried tomato pesto.

Ingredients:

1½ cups/ 400ml boiling water

1½ / 180g cups sun-dried tomatoes

1 small bulb fennel

2 cloves garlic

½ cup / 60g fresh basil leaves

2 tbs fresh oregano leaves or ½ tsp dried oregano

1 tbs lemon juice

½ tsp. sea salt

3 tbs olive oil

16 oz / 450g wheat-free pasta

Garnish options:

Sliced ripe olives, freshly ground black pepper, roasted pine-nuts, and oregano or basil sprigs

Method:

1. Pour boiling water over tomatoes; allow to sit until soft and pliable, about 5 to 8 minutes. Drain and reserve liquid. Quarter fennel bulb, remove and discard core. Thinly slice fennel.

2. Combine quarter of the fennel with sun-dried tomatoes, garlic, basil, oregano, lemon juice, salt and olive oil in a food processor or blender. Process until smooth, adding reserved tomato-soaking water a bit at a time until desired consistency is reached. Allow to rest while preparing pasta, if possible, let flavours blend 30 to 60 minutes.

3. 3. Cook and drain pasta. Combine with pesto in a large serving bowl. Toss together until evenly mixed.

To serve, mound pasta in centre of serving dish. Scatter remaining fennel over top of pasta and garnish as desired.

Variation: For a richer sauce, add up to ½ cup / 450gm pine nuts before processing, then add ¼ to 1/3rd cup / 70 to 80ml extra liquid as needed.

Pasta with Aubergine, Tomato and Chilli Sauce

Serves 4 - 6

Ingredients:

8 tbs olive oil

1 large aubergine, cut into ½ inch cubes

2 garlic cloves, finely chopped

1 fresh chilli, seeded and finely chopped

2 x 14 oz cans/ 2 x 400g chopped tomatoes

Sea salt to taste

Freshly ground black pepper to taste

3 tbs chopped parsley

Wheat-free pasta of choice –

portion measure for number of servings

Method:

1. Heat the oil in a large pan and gently fry the aubergine for about 5 minutes. Stir in the garlic

and chilli, and fry until garlic begins to colour.

2. Stir in the tomatoes, salt and pepper, and parsley. Simmer for about 30 minutes.

3. Cook the pasta, and serve with sauce poured over.

Pasta with Asparagus and Mushroom Sauce

4 servings

Ingredients:

tsp olive oil

2 garlic cloves, crushed

12 oz / 350g fresh asparagus - trimmed and cut into 1/2" diagonals

Sea salt and freshly ground black pepper

2 tbs fresh lemon juice

2 tbs minced red bell pepper

Wheat-free pasta of choice

Method:

1. Combine the mushrooms, oil, and garlic in a medium pan. Cook, covered, over low heat until the mushrooms exude their juices, 5 to 7 minutes.

2. Add the red pepper and asparagus, cook covered for 3 minutes. Uncover and cook over medium-high heat, stirring until most of the liquid is evaporated, about 3 minutes. Add salt, pepper, and lemon juice. Serve immediately.

Sun- dried Tomato Pesto

Use this sauce for a quick pasta dish. Simply cook pasta and drain, spoon in required amount of sauce and toss to mix sauce.

This basic sauce is quick and simple to make and will keep in the refrigerator for up to five days. It also makes a tasty salad dressing if you add a little more tomato juice to make it thinner.

Ingredients:

20 to 25 sun-dried tomatoes

3oz / 75g unsalted macadamia nuts

5oz / 150g fresh basil leaves remove the stems

3 garlic cloves

2 tbs tomato puree

12 fl oz / 340ml tomato juice

2 tbs balsamic vinegar

3 tsp lemon juice

4 tbs olive oil

Sea salt and freshly ground pepper

Method:

1. Put the tomatoes in a small bowl, cover with boiling water and soak for about 20 minutes or until they go soft and then drain them.

2. Put tomatoes and all other ingredients into a food processor or blender and mix till smooth. It is ready to use.

Basil Pesto

Sufficient for 2 servings with pasta as a main dish

Ingredients:

2oz / 50g fresh basil leaves

3 tbs pine nuts

4 tbs olive oil

a little lemon juice

2 garlic cloves

Sea salt to taste

Method:

Put all ingredients into a food processor or blender and blend until mixed, but not to a puree. Simply toss with fresh cooked pasta.

Coriander and Cashew Salsa

Try this tasty blend with your pasta. It also works well as a sauce with vegetables.

Ingredients:

7oz / 200g fresh cashew nuts

Large bunch of coriander

2 medium-hot red chillies -

de-seeded and chopped

Finely shredded zest of 2 limes

Juice of 2 limes

3 to 4 tbs olive oil

1 to 3 chopped garlic cloves

Sea salt

Freshly ground black pepper

Method:

Put all ingredients into a food processor or blender and blend until mixture is just combined. Needs to be a thick pouring consistency for your pasta.

Spinach and Basil Sauce

I have put in the veg ingredients as millilitres as the veg is packed down for weighing so you could use a jug to get these to the relevant ml measurement

Ingredients:

3 cups / 750ml packed spinach leaves, washed, de-stemmed, and patted dry

1½ cups / 400ml packed basil leaves, washed well, and patted dry

¾ cup / 210ml packed parsley leaves, washed well, and patted dry

½ cup / 140ml olive oil

3 tbs water

1½ tsp garlic, minced

Method:

In a blender or food processor, place all of the ingredients and puree until smooth. Add additional water, if necessary, to thin the puree so that it will drizzle off the end of a spoon.   Use as a sauce for pasta or vegetables

Pasta with Vietnamese Sauce

Ingredients:

1 lb / 450g dried rice noodles

1½ cups / 75g coriander, chopped

½ cup/ 30g sweet Thai basil leaves

2 cloves garlic, halved

½ tsp minced lemon grass

1 jalapeno pepper, seeded and minced

1 tbs fish sauce

4 tbs chopped, unsalted dry-roasted peanuts

6 tbs oil of choice

½ lime, cut into wedges

Sea salt to taste

Freshly ground black pepper to taste

Note* Many more 'high-street' supermarkets are beginning to stock ingredients for oriental dishes requiring obscure ingredients. If they do not stock them, then ask them and they may add them to their stock list.

Method:

1. 1 Soak rice noodles in a large bowl of cold water for 30 minutes. Drain and set aside.

2. Make the pesto: In a blender or food processor combine coriander, basil, garlic cloves, lemon-grass, jalapeno pepper, fish sauce and 2 tbs of peanuts. Blend until the herbs and peanuts are coarsely chopped. Then when machine is running, add the oil in a thin stream. Then add the remaining peanuts, and continue to blend until all peanuts are coarsely chopped.

3. Put the rice noodles into a large pan with ½ cup / 150ml of water over a medium-high heat. Stir until most of the water has been absorbed and the noodles are tender.

4. Add almost all of the pesto, and stir well, adding a few tbs of water if the pesto is too thick.

5. Taste the pasta and add more pesto, lime juice, fish sauce if you like. Garnish with remaining peanuts and serve immediately.

Quick Spaghetti Sauce

Serves 2 - 3

Ingredients:

3 cups / 750ml tomato sauce

1 cup / 75g mushrooms, sliced

½ cup / 50g chopped celery

¼ cup / 30g onion, shopped

¼ cup / 30g walnuts, chopped

1 large orange, peeled and roughly chopped

1 tbs garlic, chopped

Sea salt to taste

Wheat free pasta of choice

Method:

In a large pan combine all ingredients and cook on medium until vegetables are tender, about 30 minutes. Cook pasta in lightly salted water and serve immediately.

End of the main course ......

Sweets and Puddings

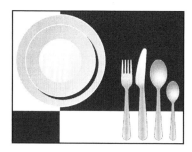

Yes! There are sweet and pudding recipes you can make without using sugar. In the introduction we talked about alternative ingredients including the alternatives for sugar. As you are obviously aware, it is very difficult to make sweets and puddings without using sugar or some type of sweetener, but I have been able to adapt the recipes in this section so they are suitable for the diet.

Yam Pie

Makes one 9 inch pie

Ingredients:

Crust:

1 cup / 100g walnuts

1 cup / 100g soaked almonds

½ cup / 125g dates, pitted

2 tbs orange juice

Method:

1. Process all nuts in a food processor, until it turns into a thick paste.

2. Add dates and keep blending for a while. Add orange juice to the mix and blend.

3. Spread mixture into a pie pan (glass preferable) evenly to form a 'crust' using your hands to press it down, and immediately set aside in the freezer.

Yam filling:

4 yams (medium to small size), peeled

1 avocado

½ cup / 125g of dates, pitted

3tbs liquid sweetener (like maple syrup)

1tsp vanilla

1tsp cinnamon

Method:

1. Cut the yams in pieces small enough to fit in a blender. Blend yams, avocado and dates in food processor.

2. Add the rest of the ingredients and mix. Then add the filling to the pie base to fill in the pie base evenly.

Options: Top with fresh shredded coconut and slices of strawberries or other fruits.

Alternative: You could try using a pie crust recipe from the baking section, then use the filling mixture above to fill the pie

Strawberry - Banana Cream Pie

Makes one 9-inch pie

Ingredients:

Crust:

¾ cup/ 100g almonds

¾ / 100g cup walnuts

½ cup / 90g dates, pitted

½ tsp cinnamon

2 tbs orange juice

Filling:

3 tbs agar-agar flakes

1/3rd cup/ 80ml apple juice

5 bananas, peeled, and cut in half length-wise

1/3rd cup/ 60g dates, pitted

½ tsp. lemon juice

1½ cups / 300g strawberries, washed, and sliced

Method:

1. Process all nuts in a food processor, until it turns into a thick paste.

2. Add dates and keep blending for a while. Add orange juice to the mix and blend.

3. Spread mixture into a pie pan (glass preferable) evenly to form a 'crust' using your hands to press it down, and immediately set aside to chill.

4. In a small bowl, place the agar-agar flakes, pour the apple juice over the flakes, and set the mixture aside for 10 minutes to allow the flakes to soften.

5. Clean out food processor, add the bananas and process for 2 minutes or until very smooth and creamy. Add the agar-agar mixture, dates, and lemon juice, and process an additional 1 minute.

6. Pour the filling over the prepared crust. Cover the top of the filling with a piece of parchment paper, place the pie in the refrigerator, and allow it to chill for 2 or more hours. Just before serving, decorate the top of the pie with the sliced strawberries.

Note: Of course you can always use other fruits that are in season for the filling.

Strawberry - Banana Pie Two – less complex

Makes one 9 inch pie

Ingredients:

Crust:

1 - 1 ½ cups / 150g to 200g soaked almonds

½ cup / 90g dates

1 tsp cinnamon

½ tsp nutmeg

¼ cup / 70ml orange juice

Filling:

3 pints / 1700ml strawberries

4 bananas

¼ cup / 70ml fresh shredded coconut

Method:

1. Freeze 2/3rds of the strawberries and 2 bananas
   Process all nuts in a food processor, until it turns into a thick paste.

2. Add dates and keep blending for a while. Add orange juice to the mix and blend.

3. Spread mixture into a pie pan (glass preferable) evenly to form a 'crust' using your hands to press it down, and immediately set aside to chill.

4. Process the frozen fruit to a sorbet consistency in a juicer. Alternatively, use a blender but let the fruit thaw a little before putting in the blender. Slice up the remaining strawberries and bananas.
   Layer the sorbet and fruit slices over the pie crust. Decorate with coconut. Keep very cool, but do not refreeze, till ready to serve.

Strawberry Pie

Makes one 9 inch pie

Another version of the non-baked pie which is quick and simple

Ingredients:

Nutty Date Crust:

½ cup / 50g walnuts

½ cup/ 50g almonds

½ cup/ 90g dates, pitted

2 tbs orange juice

Filling:

5 cups / 1000g strawberries, sliced

1 tbs maple syrup

Method:

1. Process all nuts in a food processor, until it turns into a thick paste.

2. Add dates and keep blending for a while. Add orange juice to the mix and blend.

3. Spread mixture into a pie pan (glass preferable) evenly to form a 'crust' using your hands to press it down, and immediately set aside to chill.

4. Toss the strawberries with the maple syrup. Spoon into the pie crust. Cover with waxed paper & refrigerate for 1 hour before serving.

Almond and Berry Pie

Makes one 9 inch pie

Ingredients:

Pie Crust:

1½ cups/ 120g sliced almonds

¾ cup/ 210ml sunflower seeds

½ cups / 90g dates, pitted

½ cup / 60/70g dried banana chips
or de-hydrated banana slices

½ tsp cardamom

¼ tsp cinnamon

2 tbs orange juice

Berry Filling:

2 ½ cups/ 250g blueberries

1 cup / 200g strawberries

1/3rd / 70g cup dates, pitted

½ tsp cardamom

¼ tsp cinnamon

Garnishes:

Sliced strawberries

Sliced almonds

Method:

1. In a food processor, place the almonds and sunflower seeds, and process for 2-3 minutes to form a fine meal. Add the remaining pie crust ingredients, and process for 5-7 additional minutes or until the mixture comes together.

2. Transfer the mixture to a 9-inch pie pan. Using your hands, press the mixture evenly over the bottom and up the sides of the pie pan. Place in the refrigerator and allow to chill for 20-30 minutes or until firm.

3. Wipe out the food processor for use in preparing the filling. Place all of the filling ingredients in the food processor and process for 1-2 minutes to form a smooth puree. Pour the filling into the chilled pie crust. Place the pie in the refrigerator and chill for 30-45 minutes or until filling is set and slightly firm. Decorate with a few fresh berries and sliced almonds.

Cinnamon and Raisin Bread Pudding

Makes one 8 x 12 inch pudding

Ingredients:

6 cups / 300g stale bread (non-wheat) cut into 1-inch cubes

1/3rd cup / 50g raisins

2 ½ cups / 640ml rice milk, or other non-dairy milk of choice

1 cup / 250ml apple juice

½ cup / 150ml maple syrup

1 tsp. vanilla essence

1 tsp cinnamon

½ tsp salt

¼ tsp nutmeg

Method:

1. Lightly oil a 8 x 12-inch casserole dish. Place the bread cubes in the casserole dish and scatter the raisins over the bread cubes.

2. In a small bowl, whisk together the remaining ingredients, and pour over the top of the bread cubes. Bake at 350°F/180°C for 40-45 minutes or until golden brown on top.

3. Remove from the oven and allow to sit for 10 minutes before cutting into servings. Serve warm, cold, or at room temperature, and can be served plain, or with a scoop of non-dairy ice cream or sorbet.

* Note: you can substitute other dried fruit for the raisins

Baked Apples with Blackberries

4 servings

Ingredients:

Preheat oven to 400°F/200°C

4 large eating apples

1 tbs coconut oil

8 oz / 225g blackberries

2 tbs liquid sweetener of choice

Method:

1. Wash the apples, core them, making nice wide holes, and stand them in a greased baking tray. Put a blob of coconut oil on each one.

2. Stuff the middles with all the blackberries you can cram in. Trickle with sweetener on top of each filling

3. Bake for 20 - 25 minutes, or until the apple skins are glistening and ready to burst. Serve either hot or cold.

Date and Nut Torte

A two layer Torte which is quick to prepare and ideal for parties – some of you could find this recipes a bit expensive but it would be great for a special treat

Ingredients:

1 cup / 180g pitted dates

2 cups / 300g raisins & 2 cups / 300g currants

2 cups / 200g pecans

1 lemon

2 cups / 300gm hazel nuts

2 tbs lemon juice

1 tsp lemon rind

Method:

1. Bottom layer: in food processor - blend into a fine meal the hazel nuts and raisins, and press mixture into a round shape about 1/2" thick and 8" in diameter on a plate.
2. Lemon Date frosting: in food processor or blender - blend until smooth, dates and lemon juice using water if needed to thin, stirring lemon rind into sauce at the end.
3. Frost top side of first layer of the torte with 1/2 sauce, save the rest for frosting the top
4. Top layer: in food processor: blend into a fine meal, pecans and currants, place on wax paper, make into another layer to fit on top of the first, and carefully place on top of the first frosted layer.
5. Frost the entire outside, and decorate with lemon wedges around the rim, serve or chill before serving if you wish.

Banana Cream

Makes about 1¼ pints/ 800ml

Ingredients:

2 bananas

½ pint / 300ml milk substitute

3 tbs cooked brown rice

1 level tsp grated nutmeg

Method:

Blend all ingredients in a blender until smooth. Serve at once.

Raspberry Fool

Serves 4

Ingredients:

4 cups / 500g fresh raspberries

1 to 2 cups / 250 to 500ml – creamy yoghurt (measurement depends on personal choice of consistency) use either health store alternative or your own nut based yoghurt

2 tbs granulated agar-agar

Method:

1. Briefly wizz raspberries in a blender so that raspberries form a thick puree. Add agar-agar gran-

ules, mix and leave to stand for about an hour

2. Add the yoghurt and mix together with a fork and leave to stand and chill for a while before serving.

Option: omit the agar-agar and this makes a good pouring coulis to pour over ice-cream or fresh raspberries.

Poached Pears with Fresh Strawberry Coulis

Serves 4

Ingredients:

4 firm, ripe pears, peeled, cored and halved

1 cup / 250ml apple juice concentrate or

natural fruit juice concentrate

2 cups / 470ml water

For the Coulis:

3 cups / 600g fresh strawberries

Juice of 1 lemon

2 tbs syrup from the pears

Method:

1. Place the pears flat side down in a deep roasting dish or casserole. Add the liquids, cover and cook gently on the stove until the pears are soft - approximately 40 minutes.

2. Remove the pears to a serving dish. Boil the juices left in the dish to reduce to about half the volume to form a syrup. Pour over the pears saving 2 tbs for the coulis. Chill.

3. Coulis: Mix all ingredients together in a blender until smooth. Pour over chilled pears and serve.

Baked Bananas

4 servings

Ingredients:

4 bananas

1 - 2oz / 25 – 50g coconut oil

Grated nutmeg

2 tbs raisins - well washed (optional)

2 tbs sesame seeds

Method:

Preheat oven to 400°F/200°C

1. Peel the bananas, halve them lengthways, and put them side by side in a greased fireproof dish.

2. Dot the coconut oil over them, grate a little nutmeg on top, and sprinkle with the raisins.

3. Bake for about 10 minutes, turning them over once. Remove them to a clean serving dish and scatter with sesame seeds on top.

Banana-Carob Crème Pudding

Ingredients:

6-8 medium-sized bananas
½ - 1 cup/ 60 – 120g carob, raw (to taste)
½ - 1 cup / 60 – 100g flaxseed, ground to powder (to firm up mixture – add a bit at a time)
a pinch of coconut flakes

Method:

1. Mix first three ingredients in food processor until totally smooth. Set aside in refrigerator until flax-seed powder fully gels mixture (should be firm).
2. Scoop into bowl and smooth with spatula. Can be used as pudding or pie filling.
3. Sprinkle coconut flakes in centre. The coconut flakes appear like powdered sugar.

Creamy Carob Dessert

Ingredients:

3 x 1 ½ oz / 40g bars carob confection (dairy-free, sugar-free)

2 cups / 500ml rice milk

1 tsp natural vanilla essence

1 tsp agar-agar

8 tbs cold water

Method:

1. Break up the two carob bars into a basin and stand in a saucepan of hot water.
2. Whilst melting, gently heat the milk then gradually pour onto the carob, stirring all the time. Add vanilla essence.
3. When mixed together well, remove from the heat. Put agar-agar into the cold water in a saucepan and bring to the boil. When dissolved, allow to cool then stir into the carob mix.
4. Pour through a sieve into a glass bowl or into individual glasses. Chill in the refrigerator until set like blancmange then decorate the top with the third carob bar, grated on top.

Gooseberry and Apple Mousse

Serves 4

Ingredients:

6 oz / 175g gooseberries

2 tbs apple juice

2 big crisp eating apples

2 tbs liquid sweetener of choice

Cinnamon - pinch

Nutmeg - pinch

5 oz/150 ml nut yoghurt (see Alternative Ingredients) or natural yoghurt

Method:

1. Put the gooseberries and 1 tbs of the apple juice in a pan. Cover and cook over a low heat for a couple of minutes, until the skins have split open. Put into a blender, process, and then put the puree into a large bowl. Leave to cool.
2. Peel, core, and slice the apples into a pan with 1 tbs of apple juice, a sprinkle with cinnamon, and a grating of nutmeg. Cover and cook until soft. Process in a blender and leave to cool in a bowl.
3. When both purees are cool, drain off any excess juice (save for other uses). Mix both purees together, stir in the sweetener, then whisk in the yoghurt (saving some for serving). Spoon into 4 glasses. Serve chilled decorated with a swirl of yoghurt.

Mango Pudding with nuts

Ingredients:

2 mangos

Juice of ½ lime

shredded coconut & chopped pecans, to taste

Method:

1. Peel the mangoes, then place a knife flush to one of the flat sides of the mango pit and cut all the mango away from the pit. Add lime and blend until perfectly smooth.

2. To complete the dessert, pour into dessert cups/dishes and add shredded coconut and chopped pecans to taste.

Blackberry Parfait

Serves 4

Ingredients:

1 lb / 450g blackberries

2 tbs apple juice

1 tbs sweetener of choice

½ pint / 300ml nut yoghurt (see Alternative Ingredients) or natural yoghurt – see

 introduction regards yoghurt

Method:

1. Wash the blackberries carefully - save a few for decoration. Put the fruit into a pan with the apple juice and sweetener. Heat over a very low flame until the juices run out - a few minutes only - and allow to cool.

2. When cool, blend in the yoghurt. Put in a closed, freezer-proof container, and leave in the freezer for a few hours. Take it out and give it a couple of vigorous stirs to break up any crystals that may have formed. Return to the freezer for another 3 - 4 hours. Just before serving, stir again with a fork, divide between individual glass bowls, and top each serving with blackberries.

Raspberry Frappe

Serves 4

Ingredients:

2 cups / 150g frozen raspberries

3 frozen bananas

2 tbs liquid sweetener of choice, blended with a little water if needed

Let fruit thaw a little to soften a bit.

Method:

Put all the ingredients into a food processor, process to a creamy consistency and it is ready to serve.

Rice Pudding

Serves 4

Ingredients:

1 tbs vegetable oil

2 cups / 400g cooked brown rice

½ cup / 90g chopped dates

2 tbs date sugar or other sweetener

1 tsp cinnamon

1¼ cups/ 320ml rice milk

Method:

Preheat oven to 350°F/180°C

1. Warm oil briefly in the bottom of a medium sized baking dish. Add rice, dates, date sugar, cinnamon and rice milk. Mix briefly.

2. Bake for about 30 minutes, or until done to your liking. Serve warm or cold. If pudding dries out, add more milk substitute to taste.

Brown Rice Pudding

Serves 4

Ingredients:

3 oz / 75g brown rice

32 fl oz / 950ml coconut cream or thick coconut milk

Pinch salt

6 tbs sweetener of choice

Pinch of nutmeg

3 tbs grated almonds

Method:

Preheat oven to 250°F/120°C

Stir all the ingredients together in a casserole dish, and bake uncovered for 3 hours, stirring a couple of times during the first 2 hours. Serve immediately.

Banana Ice Cream

(Using an ice cream maker)

12 servings

Ingredients:

1 cup / 100g pecans

2 large or 3 small bananas

½ cup / 150ml sweetener of choice

1½ tsp cinnamon (optional)

¾ tsp guar gum

Cold water

Method:

1. Mix pecans in blender until ground very fine. Gradually add 3 cups / 750ml very cold water. Blend on high until pecan mixture is very smooth. Add bananas, sweetener, cinnamon, and guar gum. Blend until mixture is very smooth.

2. Pour approximately half of mixture into a 2-quart / 2250ml ice cream maker. Blend 1 cup / 250ml cold water with mixture left in blender container. Pour into ice cream maker and stir to mix with the first batch. Freeze according to manufacturer's instructions,

3. When ice cream is finished, cover and store in freezer for a couple of hours before serving so it will firm up.

Carob Ice Cream

(Using an ice cream maker)

8 servings

4 cups / 1 litre container of carob flavoured rice drink

¼ cup / 70ml sweetener of choice

2 tbs vegetable oil

¾ tsp guar gum

Method:

1. Chill rice beverage for several hours in the refrigerator. Combine 3 cups / 750ml of the rice beverage, sweetener, oil, and guar gum in blender container. Blend until mixture is very smooth. Pour approximately half of the mixture into a 2-quart / 2250ml ice cream maker. Add the rest of the 1 litre container of rice drink into the blender, and mix again. Pour into ice-cream maker and stir well to mix. Freeze according to manufacturer's instructions.

2. When ice cream is finished, cover and store in the freezer for a couple of hours before serving so it will firm up.

Strawberry & Coconut Ice-cream

Try to find a good thick creamy coconut milk for this recipe, as they do vary in thickness depending on the make. A watery coconut milk will produce more of a sorbet rather than a rich ice cream.

Ingredients:

1 lb / 450g strawberries

450ml / 2 cups thick coconut milk

Method:

1. Halve the strawberries, place on a baking tray and freeze uncovered. Place the coconut milk in the refrigerator until very cold.

2. Place the coconut milk in a food processor. It is a god idea to wrap a tea towel round the processor to prevent splashing when the strawberries are added

3. Switch on the processor and add the frozen strawberries in through the funnel. Process the mixture until smooth. You will need to remove the lid and use a spatula to help combine the ingredients if they are not processing smoothly. Serve immediately.

The Simplest Ice-Cream

Take fresh, raw, ripe fruit like mangos, bananas, papaya. This does not work with watery fruit like strawberries or raspberries. Peel and slice your chosen fruit, and store slices in plastic bag or other suitable container, and freeze.

Then when you want to make up your 'ice-cream', remove from freezer and allow fruit to partially thaw. The fruit should not fully thaw; it should still have ice crystals in it.

Put partially thawed fruit in a blender, and puree. The result is an ice cream substitute that is 100% raw fruit, delicious, and better than any commercial ice cream.

You could try adding carob with banana, for a Carob and Banana 'ice-cream'.

Fruit Salad

Do not forget the simplest of sweets - the fruit salad. Choose fruits which are in season as they will be grown in your area and you can buy local organic produce. Peel and chop up all your fruit and pour fresh fruit juice over the top. You can dress it up with coconut flakes, a few chopped nuts and serve with some organic Greek yoghurt or the simple ice-cream recipe previous.

Onto the baking section next ......

Get those 'pinnies' out and roll up your sleeves!

Baking, Breads and Pie Crusts

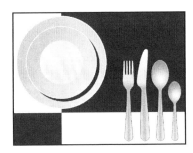

Being on a diet for Endometriosis requires the elimination of wheat from your diet. This does not mean that you cannot have breads, cakes and pastries. It simply means using alternative flours, and there are quite a few to choose from.

When it comes to baking and bread recipes for a diet for Endometriosis, it is very hard to eliminate all ingredients that should be avoided, especially the use of eggs or sweetener, but I have put these recipes together stating the use of alternative ingredients.

If you prefer to use standard ingredients regarding eggs or sweetener, then the amounts you will be ingesting per serving will be minimal.

These recipes use a variety of flours, some of them totally *Gluten free*, others with low levels of gluten. Egg substitute can be used instead of fresh eggs. (See 'Substitute Ingredients' section)   If you are going to use fresh eggs, make sure you use free-range, organic eggs.

The use of sweetening in everyday baking is by sugars of different types. There is also a list of alternative sweeteners in the 'Substitute Ingredients' section.

You can always experiment with these recipes. You can try different types of oil, and different types of sweeteners.

Alternatives to Wheat Flour

Many grains can be used to replace wheat. I have included most of the *Gluten free* alternative flours you can use, but have listed other flours that you need to omit for the Endometriosis diet.

Here is a basic list of flours and their properties:

Amaranth flour - *Gluten free* - Unrelated to wheat - Amaranth flour is made from the seed of the Amaranth plant, which is a leafy vegetable. Amaranth seeds are very high in protein, which makes it a nutritious flour for baking.

Barley flour - *Small amount of gluten* - Related to wheat so should be rotated - Barley only contains a small amount of gluten, so is rarely used to make bread, with the exception of unleavened bread. It has a slightly nutty flavour, and can be used to thicken or flavour soups or stews. Blended with other alternative flours it is also fairly versatile for cakes, biscuits, pastry, dumplings etc.

Brown rice flour - *Gluten free* - Related to wheat so should be rotated - Brown rice flour is heavier than its relative, white rice flour. It is milled from unpolished brown rice so it has a higher nutritional value than white, and as it contains the bran of the brown rice it has higher fibre content. This also means that it has a noticeable texture, a bit grainy.

Buckwheat flour - *Gluten free* - Unrelated to wheat - It does have a slight nutty taste, which will sometimes come out in recipes depending on the other ingredients, and the texture will also contribute to a heavier product than recipes made with white rice flour. It is not often used completely on its own because of its heavier nature. Bulk buying is not recommended as it is better used when fresh, store in an airtight container.

139

Corn-flour - *Gluten free* - is milled from corn into a fine, white powder, and is used for thickening recipes and sauces. It has a bland taste, and therefore is used in conjunction with other ingredients that will impart flavour to the recipe. It also works very well when mixed with other flours, for example when making fine batters for tempura. Some types of corn-flour are milled from wheat but are labelled wheaten corn-flour. Alternative name: corn-starch.

Chickpea flour - *Gluten free* - Unrelated to wheat - This is ground from chick peas and has a strong slightly nutty taste. It is not generally used on its own. Nutritious but expensive

Millet flour - *Gluten free* - Related to wheat so should be rotated - Comes from the grass family, and is used as a cereal in many African and Asian countries. It can be used to thicken soups and make flat breads and griddle cakes. Because it lacks any form of gluten it's not suited to many types of baking.

Oat flour - *Small amount of gluten* - Ground from oats. Care also needs to be taken to ensure that it is sourced from a non-wheat contaminating process.

Potato flour - *Gluten free* - This flour should not be confused with potato starch flour. Potato flour has a strong potato flavour and is a heavy flour so a little goes a long way. Bulk buying is not recommended unless you are using it on a very regular basis for a variety of recipes as it does not have a very long shelf life.

Quinoa flour - *Gluten free* - Unrelated to wheat - Quinoa is related to the plant family of spinach and beets. It has been used for over 5,000 years as a cereal, and the Incas called it the mother seed. Quinoa provides a good source of vegetable protein and it is the seeds of the quinoa plant that are ground to make flour.

Rye flour - *Contains small amount of gluten* - Closely related to wheat so not suitable for endometriosis diet - Rye flour is a strongly flavoured flour, dark in colour.

Sorghum flour - *Gluten free* - Not related to wheat - Ground from sorghum grain, which is similar to millet. The flour is used to make porridge or flat unleavened breads. It is an important staple in Africa and India. This flour stores well under normal temperatures. However, due to the stress this plant can undergo during growing by high temperatures and drought it can contain toxic levels of cyanide and/or nitrates at later stages in growth, therefore it is not a sources of flour I would recommend.

Spelt flour - Related to wheat so not advised for the endometriosis diet

Teff flour - *Gluten free* - Distantly related to wheat so fine for the endometriosis diet - Teff comes from the grass family, and is a tiny cereal grain native to northern Africa. It is ground into flour and used to prepare injera, which is a spongy, slightly sour flat bread. It is now finding a niche in the health food market because it is very nutritious.

White rice flour - *Gluten free* - This flour is milled from polished white rice so it is very bland in taste, and not particularly nutritious. White rice flour is ideal for recipes that require a light texture, for example herb dumplings. It can be used on its own for a variety of recipes and has a reasonable shelf life, as long as it is stored in an airtight container to avoid it absorbing moisture from the air.

Millet, oats, rice, barley and teff are grains in the same botanical family as wheat. This means they should be rotated by wheat sensitive people. All these grains are available as flour and each has different characteristics.

Millet and brown rice flour usually have a grainy texture. When used alone in baked goods they require a binder, such as egg or arrowroot.

Oat flour is exceptionally fine and sticky and does not behave like wheat flour, but it is sweet and has other desirable characteristics. Oat flour makes very good pancakes, cookies and muffins.

Barley flour is fine, and relatively tasteless. It is easy to substitute for wheat flour in most situations. As is does not have sufficient gluten, a binding agent is required to prevent it from crumbling.

Teff flour is expensive, but can be used as a substitute for some wheat flour recipes. It makes good pie crust and is best mixed with other flours because of its heavy texture.

Amaranth and quinoa flour sometimes have a bitter taste and also need to be stored in the refrigerator. Both flours lack gluten so need a binding agent.

Buckwheat flour is available in two grades - light and dark. The dark is more commonly available, but its usefulness is limited by its strong taste. Dark buckwheat is good in pancakes. Light buckwheat is a good substitute for wheat flour. It has the same colour and texture, and even has enough gluten that helps dough stick together, so that an additional binding agent is not required.

Chick-pea flour is readily available and can be used in muffins, cookies, and pancakes but is rather expensive. If you want to avoid soy flour, and soy is used as only part of the flour content of the recipe, substitute with chick-pea flour.

Pancakes

Oatmeal Pancakes

Low in gluten

Preheat oven to 350°F/180°C

Ingredients:

¾ cup / 95g quick oats

¼ tsp baking soda

1½ cups/ 390ml water

½ cup/ 65g ground oats

1 tsp sweetener of choice

1 tsp baking powder

½ tsp salt

Beaten together:

3 tsp oil

2 tsp water

1 tsp baking powder

Method:

1. Combine oats, baking soda and 1½ cups / 390ml water; let stand for 5 minutes.
2. Combine ground oats, sugar, 1 tsp baking powder and salt. Add to this pre-blended oil, water and baking powder and beat well.
3. Pour 1/4 cup / 70ml batter for each pancake onto a hot greased griddle. Bake at 350°F/180°C to a golden brown, turning once. Makes 10 pancakes.

Rice Potato Pancakes

Gluten free

Ingredients:

½ cup / 65g rice flour

1/3rd cup/ 45g potato flour

¼ tsp salt

2 tsp liquid sweetener

½ tsp baking powder

1/3rd to ½ cup water / 80 – 150ml

Beaten together:

1 ½ tsp oil

1 ½ tsp water

1 tsp baking powder

Method:

1. Sift dry ingredients together. Beat in 1/3rd to ½ cup / 80 – 150ml water. Beat in the mixture of oil, water and baking powder.

2. Cook on a hot greased griddle, using about ¼ cup/ 70ml batter for each pancake. Turn once.

(This recipe works really well, does not stick and tastes very like pancakes made with wheat flour.)

Gram Flour Pancakes

Gluten free

Makes 24 x four inch cakes

Ingredients:

¾ cup / 100 g gram/chickpea flour

½ tsp salt

350 ml iced water

Oil for frying

Method:

1. Mix flour, salt (and spices if required) together. Gradually add iced water until you get a smooth batter.

2. Heat a little oil in a pan, add a quarter of the batter and cook until the edges are crispy and brown, and the top has dried out. Serve with filling of your choice.

3. Continue to cook rest of mixture, keeping warm in oven till ready

Amaranth Pancakes/Flatbread

Gluten free

Ingredients:

½ cup / 65g almond flour

1 cup / 125g amaranth flour

½ arrowroot starch

½ tsp baking soda

¼ tsp sea salt

1 tsp ground cinnamon

1 - 2 tbs maple syrup

1& ½ cups / 400ml water

2 tbs fresh lemon juice

2 tsp cream of tartar

2 tbs light oil

Method:

1. Combine liquids in a blender; blend for about 10 seconds

2. In another bowl blend together all dry ingredients

3. Mix wet and dry ingredients together in mixing bowl

4. Cook pancakes on preheated, un-greased, griddle or fry pan. When bubbly and brown, turn.

Serve immediately

As batter thickens you may need to add another tablespoon or two of water to keep cakes thin (should be no more than ¼ inch thick)

Muffins and Buns

All Round Muffin/Buns

Gluten free

12 muffins/buns

This is a very versatile muffin recipe. Any of the alternative flours can be used. Choose from buckwheat, amaranth, quinoa, or brown rice flour to make this Gluten free. Take your choice of several kinds of fruit, nuts and moistener.

Ingredients:

½ cup / 65g each of amaranth, quinoa,

and light buckwheat flour

2 tbs arrowroot powder

2 tsp baking powder

1 tsp cinnamon

¼ tsp salt

½ to 1 cup / 50 – 100g chopped nuts

(pecans, walnuts, brazil nuts)

3 tbs milk substitute or fruit juice

1 tbs light oil

1 tbs sweetener of choice (optional)

1 large ripe banana mashed,

or ½ to ¾ cup/ 25 – 50g of shredded courgette

1 egg (optional)

Method:

Preheat oven to 425°F/220°C

1. Grease a muffin/bun tin with vegetable oil. Combine flours, arrowroot, baking powder, cinnamon, salt, and nuts in a bowl. Make a well in the dry ingredients and add milk/fruit juice, oil, sweetener, mashed banana or courgette and egg. Mix lightly, adding more liquid if needed to moisten flour. More liquid will be required if the egg of sweetener is omitted. Add 3 tbs, then mix. If necessary, add more liquid, 2 tbs at a time, until the flour is moistened. Dough should be fairly stiff.

2. Divide the dough evenly among 12 muffin cups. Bake about 12 to 15 minutes. Immediately after removal from oven, loosen muffins and turn them out to cool.

Carob Buckwheat Muffins/Buns

Gluten free

Ingredients:

1/3rd cup / 35g pecan nuts

1 cup/ 250ml boiling water

¼ cup / 70ml walnut oil

¼ cup/ 70ml maple syrup

1 cup / 130g buckwheat flour

1/3rd / 45g cup carob powder

½ cup / 65g coarsely chopped pecans

2 tsp baking powder

¾ tsp ground cinnamon

¼ tsp baking soda

2 eggs or egg substitute

1 tsp pure vanilla extract (optional)

Method:

1. Grind pecans to a fine powder in a blender, add water, and blend for 30 seconds, add oil and maple syrup, blend again. Allow to cool to lukewarm.

2. Combine flour, carob, chopped pecans, baking powder, cinnamon and baking soda in a large bowl. Mix well.

3. When the liquid mixture has cooled to lukewarm, blend in the eggs and vanilla.

4. Pour liquid mixture into the flour bowl. Mix to moisten all dry ingredients. Bake in muffin cases at 400°F/200°C till golden on top

Carob Muffins 2

Gluten free

Ingredients:

1 cup / 130g chick pea flour

1 tbs carob powder

1 tbs arrowroot powder

1 ½ tsp baking powder

Dash salt

½ cup / 150ml milk substitute

2 tbs maple syrup (optional)

2 tbs light oil

Method:

Preheat oven to 350°F/180°C

1. Grease a muffin/bun tin with vegetable oil. Combine flour, carob, arrowroot, baking powder and salt in a medium mixing bowl. Combine milk, maple syrup and oil in a pan. Heat liquid ingredients briefly (about 2 to 3 mins) to blend ingredients. If maple syrup is omitted, heating is not necessary, but a little more liquid may be needed. Add liquid ingredients to flour mixture and mix briefly.

2. Divide the dough evenly among 6 muffin cups and bake for 15 to 18 minutes. Immediately after removal from oven, loosen muffins with a fork and turn out to cool.

Oat Bran Muffins

Small amount of gluten

12 muffins

Ingredients:

1 & ¼ cups / 160g oat bran

1 cup / 130g oat flour

1 tbs arrowroot powder

½ tsp cinnamon

¼ tsp salt

¼ cup / 40g currant or raisins (optional)

¼ cup / 30g chopped pecans or other nuts

1 cup / 250ml apple

or pineapple juice, or milk substitute

2 tbs light oil

2 tbs liquid sweetener (optional)

Method:

Preheat oven to 425°F/220°C

1. Grease a muffin tin with vegetable oil. Combine oat bran, flour, arrowroot, baking powder, cinnamon, salt, currants, and nuts in a medium bowl. Combine juice, oil, and sweetener in a small pan. Heat briefly (about 2 to 3 mins). (If sweetener is omitted, heating is not necessary, but a little more liquid may be required). Add to dry ingredients and mix just until the dry ingredients are moistened.

2.   Divide the dough evenly among the 12 muffin cups and bake for 15 to 18 minutes. Immediately after removal from oven, loosen muffins and turn out to cool. Variation: Add a mashed banana for even moister muffins. Reduce liquid to 2/3rds cup / 170ml

Apple Amaranth Muffins

Gluten free

12 muffins - The apple in these muffins makes them moist and special.

Ingredients:

1½ cups / 190g amaranth flour

2 tbs arrowroot powder

2 tsp baking powder

1 tsp cinnamon

Dash salt

1 cup / 100g grated apple

½ cup / 110g chopped walnuts or other nuts

¾ cup / 210g apple juice or milk substitute

¼ cup/ 70ml light oil

¼ cup / 70ml liquid sweetener (optional)

1 egg (optional)

Method:

Preheat oven to 400°F/200°C

1. Grease a muffin tin with vegetable oil. Combine flour, arrowroot, baking powder, cinnamon, salt, grated apple, and nuts in a medium mixing pan. Mix juice, oil, and sweetener in a pan. Heat briefly (about 2 to 3 mins) to blend ingredients. (This step is not necessary if sweetener is omitted). Add egg to this mixture, if desired. Stir and then pour into flour mixture, and mix together quickly. If egg or sweetener is omitted, batter may be too stiff. Add just enough liquid to moisten dry ingredients.

2. Divide the dough evenly among the 12 muffin cups and bake 15 to 18 minutes. Immediately after removal from oven, loosen muffins with a fork and turn out to cool.

Cookies

Quick Oat and Raisin Cookies

Small amount of gluten

Makes 16 - 18

Ingredients:

3 cups / 380g oats

1½ cups 190g rice flour

1 cup / 150g raisins

1 cup / 125g chopped nuts of your choice

4 tbs olive oil

1 tbs apple juice concentrate

Apple juice to mix

Method:

Preheat oven to 370°F/180°C

1. Mix all ingredients together well, using just enough apple juice to make a mixture with a soft 'dropping' consistency.
2. Divide mixture into flattened rough cookie shapes on oiled baking sheets
3. Bake for about 20 minutes, remove from oven and place on wire rack to cool.

Date and Banana Cookies

Small amount of gluten

Ingredients:

Makes about 18 to 20

Preheat oven to 375°F/190°C

½ cup / 90g dried dates, finely chopped

2/3rds / 75g cup walnuts, finely chopped

3 medium bananas, mashed

2 cups / 250g oats

½ cup / 140ml olive oil

1 tsp vanilla essence

Method:

Mix everything together really well and put tablespoons of the mixture onto an oiled baking sheet. Flatten them down a bit and bake for about 20 minutes until golden.

This makes a lot of cookies and they freeze well for later.

Cakes
Time for some treats for endo gals!!

Banana and Hazelnut Cake

Gluten free

Makes 1 loaf

Preheat oven to 350°F/180°C

Ingredients:

3 cups / 450g ripe bananas, mashed

½ cup / 65g hazelnuts, chopped

½ cup / 140ml sunflower or olive oil

4 oz raisins

1 cup / 130g rice flour

1 tsp almond essence or vanilla essence

Method:

Mix all ingredients together well and turn into a greased 1lb/ 450g loaf tin. Bake for 50 to 60 minutes. Let cool in the tin before serving.

Carrot Fruit Cake

Gluten free - This is a no cook recipe

Ingredients:

Cake:

1 cup / 250ml dried figs, soaked – this is wet measurement because of soaking

1 cup / 250ml raisins, soaked – also in wet measurement - use a measuring jug

½ cup / 225g dates (stones removed)

4 cups s/ 150g shredded carrots

3 cups / 750ml soaked nuts (almonds, walnut, or cashews) – using wet measurement as above

½ teaspoon each: ginger, cloves, cardamom

Topping:

½ cup / 110g dates

½ cup / 50g cashews

½ cup / 150ml soaking water

Method:

1.   Soak figs, raisins and dates in 3 ½ cups / 900ml of water for one hour, reserving liquid. Soak nuts in 5 cups / 1200ml of water for 8-12 hours. Drain, rinse and drain nuts again.

2.   Place nut in food processor and chop finely, place in large bowl. Add figs, raisins, dates and spices to processor and process until smooth. Pour mixture into bowl with the nuts. Mix well.

3.   Add carrots, mix thoroughly. Form mixture into desired shape.

4.   Process dates, cashews and soaking water until smooth. Spread on top of the cake.

Banana and Date Cake

Gluten free – if you choose a Gluten free flour

Ingredients:

1½ cups / 190g all-purpose wheat free flour

2 tsp baking powder

7 or 8 large dates, soaked

½ cup / 150ml water

2 very ripe bananas, mashed

1 cup / 250ml of rice milk

½ cup / 140ml light oil

1 tablespoon of vinegar

Method:

Preheat oven to 380°F/190°C

1. Mix the flour and baking powder. Liquidise the soaked dates in the half cup of water until fairly thick and smooth. Add the date mixture to the flour along with the rice milk, oil and bananas.

2. Mix well - you may need to add a little more water or rice milk as wheat free flours do vary greatly and tend to absorb more liquid than wheat. Add the vinegar at the last minute and then pour into 9"/18cm cake tin and bake for about 40 minutes or until cooked through.

Apple Layer Cake

Small amount of gluten

A moist cake using rice flour. Nice served as a pudding with nut yoghurt.

Ingredients:

1½ cups / 190g rice flour

¼ cup / 30g oat flour

½ cup / 140ml sweetener of choice

1 tsp wheat free raising agent

2 large eating apples (peeled, cored and thinly sliced)

1 cup / 250ml water

¼ cup / 70ml of apple juice

2 tbs of light oil

A few drops of vanilla extract (optional)

Dash of vinegar

Method:

Preheat oven to 365°F/185°C

Mix the dry ingredients together then add the water, juice, oil, vanilla and mix well. Add the vinegar and stir. Pour half the cake batter into a greased square cake tin (9x9 inches or 20x20 cm approx. works well). Spread the apple slices evenly over the batter and then top with the remaining mixture and bake in oven for about 40 minutes or until firm.

Orange Pineapple Cake

Small amount of gluten

Ingredients:

2½ cups / 320g Barley or Kamut flour

2 tbs baking powder

1 tbs oil - plus

½ cup / 140ml oil

½ cup / 140ml maple syrup

¾ cup / 210ml orange juice and ¾ ml cup pineapple juice

½ cup / 150ml orange pieces, chopped small

½ cup / 200g pineapple chunks, chopped small

½ cup / 75g coconut, shredded

½ cup / 150ml raisins, pre-soaked in hot- water and drained

Method:

Preheat oven to 325°F/160°C

1. Oil bottom and sides of a cake pan with 1 tbs oil and line cake pan with wax paper. In medium bowl thoroughly mix flour and baking powder.

2. In 2nd bowl whisk together remaining ingredients, adding in fruit and raisins last. Thoroughly stir wet mixture into dry mixture to create batter.

3. Pour batter into cake pan. Bake in the oven for about 30 minutes or until fork or toothpick comes out clean. Let cake cool before removing wax paper.
    Note: Wheat-free cakes tend to be a little more crumbly than wheat cakes. This cake is also a little heavy so the wax paper will make it easier to remove from the pan.

Jamaican Banana Bread

More of a cake than a bread

Gluten free

Ingredients:

225g / 8oz peeled bananas

125ml / ½ cup water

1 egg or egg replacer

60ml / ¼ cup sunflower oil

90g / 3oz / 9 tbsp rice flour

90g / 3oz / 9 tbsp polenta flour

60g / 2oz / 6 tbsp potato flour

4 tsp baking powder

I heaped tsp ground cinnamon

½ tsp allspice

½ tsp grated nutmeg

60g / 2oz / 2/3rds cup walnuts

60g / 3oz / ½ cup raisins

Method:

Preheat oven 170c / 325F

1. Place the bananas, water, egg and oil in food processor and process till smooth. Add the flours, baking powder and spices and process again. If you do not have a processor, mash the bananas till smooth, then mix in the water, egg, oil, flours, baking powder and spices.

2. Break the walnuts into small pieces and add to the mixture along with the raisins. Mix in. If using food processor, process for 10 seconds until the walnuts are raisins are mixed in but not broken up.

3. Place the mixture in a greased and lined 1 lb loaf tin. Bake for 45 minutes or until brown on top and firm to touch.

4. Cool for 5 minutes in the tin and turn out onto wire tray. Eat within 3 days or freeze

Breads

You may, or may not want to make your own bread but on your good days you may feel up to it. I have included a couple of recipes here so that you have the option.

Fortunately many health shops now sell wheat free/Gluten free ready-made breads.

Grain Free Boston Brown Bread

Gluten free

Ingredients:

1 & 1/8th cups / 145g amaranth flour

¼ cup / 30g arrowroot

1 tsp baking soda

½ tsp powdered ginger

½ cup / 75g currants

½ cup / 100g Brazil nuts

¾ cup / 210ml boiling un-sweetened

fruit juice or water

¼ cup/ 70ml molasses

1 tsp lemon juice

Method:

1. Oil a 1lb / 450g baking tin. Fill a Dutch oven or stock pot with about 5 inches of water. Bring water to the boil.

2. In a large bowl combine the flour, arrowroot, baking soda and ginger, stir in the currants.

3. In a blender grind the nuts to a fine powder, add the juice or water and blend for 20 seconds. If the ingredients in the blender do not reach the one cup mark, add a little more liquid. With the blender running low add the molasses and lemon juice.

4. Pour the liquid mixture into the flour bowl, stir quickly to blend, do not over-mix.

5. Transfer to the prepared mould or can. Cover with a square of foil or wax paper; tie the wax paper securely with a piece of string. Place the mould in the boiling water, cover the pot tightly and steam for 2 hours over a medium low heat. Don't remove cover during this time. Remove the mould from pot and cool for 15 minutes. When cool, remove bread

Quinoa Quick Bread

Gluten-free

A quick and easy recipe

Ingredients:

1 cup / 130g quinoa flour

½ cup / 60g arrowroot

¾ tbs baking soda

½ tsp Xanthan gum

1/3rd cup / 45g oat flour

½ tsp sea salt

1½ tsp baking powder

2 tsp egg replacement

1½ cups / 400ml water

¼ cup / 70ml olive oil

Method:

Preheat oven to 375ºF/190ºC lightly oil a bread loaf tin and set aside

1. In a large mixing bowl blend all the dry ingredients together: add egg replacement, water and olive oil. Mix well

2. Bake for 20 mins then lower oven temperature to 325°F/160°C and bake for 10 more minutes

3. When cooked, place loaf on wire rack to cool before slicing

Flat Bread

Small amount of gluten

This flat bread goes well with soups, beans, stews - any hearty main dish

Ingredients:

¾ cup / 90g brown rice flour

¾ cup / 90g barley flour

2 tbs arrowroot powder

1½ tsp baking powder

1 tsp caraway seeds (optional)

¼ tsp salt

2 tbs light oil

1 tbs sweetener (optional)

1 egg (optional)

Approx. ½ cup / 150ml milk substitute

Method:

Preheat oven to 350°F/180°C

1. Mix dry ingredients in a medium bowl. Add oil, sweetener, egg, and milk to flour mixture. Start with a little less than ½ cup liquid, and add more until you get a stiff batter. If egg and/or sweetener is omitted, you may need to add a little more liquid.

2. Transfer dough to a greased baking sheet and shape into a flat round shape 1 to 1 ½ inches thick. Bake about 25 mins. Cut the bread into 8 wedge-shaped pieces for serving. Remove from baking sheet and cool on a wire rack.

Rice-Quinoa Batter Yeast Bread

Gluten free

A savoury loaf ideal for go with soups and casseroles

Makes one loaf

Ingredients:

2 tbs flax seed

1 tbs active dry yeast

2 tbs sweetener

1½ cups / 180g brown rice flour

1½ cups 190g quinoa flour

¼ cup / 30g arrowroot powder

1 tbs psyllium husk

1 tsp caraway seeds

½ tsp dried basil

½ tsp dill weed

½ tsp garlic powder

3 tbs light oil

1½ tsp salt

Method:

1. Boil flax seed in 1½ cups / 400ml water for 10 mins. Remove from heat and allow to cool.

2. Measure ½ cup / 150ml warm water, yeast, and sweetener into a small bowl. Briefly stir and let soak for 10 to 15 mins to soften yeast.

3. Meanwhile, measure rice flour, quinoa flour, arrowroot, psyllium, and spices into a medium mixing bowl and mix together. When flax mixture has cooled to lukewarm, pour it into large bowl for electric mixer. Add 1 cup / 250ml of the flour and the yeast mixture and mix on low speed. Add the vegetable oil and salt and mix well on medium speed. Gradually add most of the rest of the flour, reserving ½ cup/ 250ml. Beat at medium speed for 3 mins. Scraping sides of the bowl often with a spatula. Mix in the last half cup of flour with a spoon.

4. Cover bowl and place in a warm (set very low) oven to rise for 1 to 1 ½ hours, or until double in bulk. Grease a 9 x 5 inch bread tin, and dust lightly with flour. Fill pan with bread mixture.

5. Put back in warm oven, heating it a few seconds if it is too cool. The dough will rise very quickly. After 10 to 15 mins., when the dough is just above the top of the pan, turn the oven up to 350°F/180°C and cook for 50 minutes. Remove from pan immediately and cool on wire rack.

Note: You can vary the herbs as desired.

Barley Batter Yeast Bread

Small amount of gluten

Barley flour is usually finely ground and light in colour, so barley bread has a light texture and colour and it tastes good.

Makes 1 loaf

Ingredients:

2 tbs flax seed

2 tbs liquid sweetener

1 tbs active dry yeast

3 ½ cups / 450g barley flour

¼ cup / 30g arrowroot powder

3 tbs light oil

1½ tsp salt

Method:

1. Boil flax seed in 1 ½ cups / 400ml of water for 10 mins. Remove from heat and allow to cool slightly

2. Measure ½ cup / 150ml warm water (about 110°F/40°C), sweetener, and yeast into a small bowl. Stir briefly and let soak for 10 to 15 mins. To soften yeast

3. Meanwhile, measure barley flour and arrowroot into a medium mixing bowl and mix together. When flax mixture has cooled to lukewarm, pour into large bowl for electric mixer. Add 1 cup / 250ml of the barley flour and the yeast mixture and mix on a low speed. Add the oil and salt and mix well on medium speed. Gradually add most of the rest of the barley flour, reserving ¾ cup/ 210ml. Beat at medium speed for 3 mins., scraping the sides of the bowl often with a spatula. Mix in the last ¾ cup / 210ml of flour with a spoon.

4. Cover bowl and place in a warm oven (85 degrees) oven for about 1 to 1 ½ hours, or until double in bulk. Remove from oven and stir with a wooden spoon for 1 minute. Grease a 9 x 5 inch bread pan, and dust lightly with barley flour. Fill pan with bread mixture.

5. Put back in oven, heating it for a few seconds if it too cool. The dough will rise very quickly. After about 10 to 12 minutes, when the dough is just above the top of the pan, turn the oven on to 350°F/180°C and cook for 50 minutes. Remove from pan immediately, and cool on wire rack.

Buckwheat Batter Yeast Bread

Gluten free

Makes 1 loaf

Buckwheat in not related to wheat. This loaf is very tasty, slices nicely, and makes good sandwiches. Double the recipe if you wish as this bread freezes well

Ingredients:

½ cup / 150ml milk substitute or water

2 tbs liquid sweetener

1 tbs active dry yeast

2 ½ cups / 320ml light buckwheat flour

3 tbs light oil

¾ tsp salt

Method:

1. Measure ¾ cup / 210ml warm water (about 110°F/40°C), warm the milk substitute, add 1 table spoon sweetener, and yeast into a large bowl of an electric mixer. Stir briefly and let soak for 10 to 15 mins. - to soften yeast.

2. When the yeast is bubbly, gradually mix 1 cup / 250ml of the buckwheat flour into the yeast mixture with the electric mixer on low speed. Add oil, 1 tablespoon sweetener, and salt to the bread dough and mix. Gradually add all but ½ cup / 65g of flour. Beat at medium speed for 3 mins., scraping the sides of the bowl often with a spatula. Mix in the last ½ cup of flour with a spoon.

3. Cover bowl and place in a warm oven (110°F/25°C) to rise for 1 to 1½ hours, or until doubled in bulk. Remove from oven and stir with a wooden spoon for 1 minute. Grease a 9 x 5 inch bread pan will and dust with buckwheat flour. The dough is very sticky, so do not skimp on this step. Fill pan with bread mixture.

4. Put back in the warm oven, heating it a few seconds if it is too cool. The dough will rise quickly. After 12 to 15 mins., when the dough is just above the top of the pan, turn the oven on to 350°F/180°C and cook for 40 minutes. Let cool for 10 mins. before removing from pan. Cool on a wire rack.

Fruit Breads

Banana Bread

Gluten free

Makes 1 loaf

Ingredients:

1 ¼ cups / 200g millet flour

½ cup/ 60g arrowroot powder

2 tsp baking powder

dash salt

½ cup / 50g chopped pecans

¼ cup / 70ml oil

¼ cup / 70ml maple syrup or other sweetener

1 egg (optional)

2 medium ripe bananas, mashed

Method:

Preheat oven to 350°F/180°C

1. Grease a 9 x 5 inch bread tin with vegetable oil and dust well with millet flour. Mix millet flour, arrowroot, baking powder salt and pecans in a bowl. Mix oil, maple syrup, egg, and bananas in a bowl.

2. Add liquid ingredients to dry ingredients and mix well. Spread batter in the tin and bake about 50 minutes or until a toothpick inserted in the middle comes out clean. Let cool 10 minutes before removing from the tin.

Options: To substitute the egg - add I tablespoon psyllium seed husk powder to the dry ingredients, and 3 tablespoons water to the liquid ingredients.

Banana - Orange Nut Bread

Small amount of gluten

1 loaf

Ingredients:

2 oranges, enough for 1 cup juice and 1 tbs grated peel

1 ripe banana, mashed

¼ cup / 70ml vegetable oil

1/3rd cup / 80ml liquid sweetener

1 egg or egg substitute

2 cups / 250g barley flour

2 tbs arrowroot powder

2 tsp baking powder

¼ tsp salt

¾ cup / 80g chopped walnuts, almonds, or pecans

Method:

Preheat oven to 350°F/180°C

1. Grease a 9 x 5 inch bread tin with vegetable oil and dust well with flour. Grate the peel from the oranges and extract the juice. Put peel and juice in blender container. Add oil, sweetener, and egg. Blend long enough to mix well, and then add the banana. Blend just enough to combine ingredients.

2. Combine flour, arrowroot, baking powder, salt and nuts in a mixing bowl. Pour the liquid ingredients over the dry ingredients and mix well. Pour into tin and bake for 60 to 65 minutes.

Breakfast cakes

Potato Cakes

Gluten free

Ingredients:

½ lb / 225g cooked potatoes

2 oz / 50g gluten-free flour of choice

3 tbs oil

¼ tsp salt

¼ tsp baking powder

A little milk if required for binding or milk substitute

Method:

1. Put the flour, salt and baking powder into a bowl, mixing well, then add the sieved potatoes and the oil. Mix to a smooth dough, adding a little milk if required.

2. Place on a floured board and knead, shape and cut into triangles, cook on a hot greased griddle until brown on both sides.

Oatmeal Patty Cakes

Small amount of gluten

Ingredients:

1¼ cups / 320ml water

2/3rds / 120g cup rolled oats

¼ cup/ 40g raisins

¼ tsp cinnamon

2 tsp walnut oil

2 tsp apple butter

2 tbs chopped pecans

Method:

1. Combine the water, oats, raisins, and cinnamon in a saucepan, bring to the boil, then reduce heat, and simmer for 5 minutes. Stir frequently, stir in oil and leave to stand for 5 minutes.

2. Divide the mixture into 2 large or 4 small mounds on a plate, flatten each mound into a patty with the back of spoon, spread the top of each with apple butter and sprinkle with nuts.

Buckwheat Breakfast Cake

Gluten free

Ingredients:

1 & 2/3rds cups / 420ml water

½ cup / 75g raisins

½ lb / 225g pitted dates, chopped.

1/3rd cup/ 80ml oil

2 tsp lemon juice

1 cup/ 130g buckwheat flour

1 cup / 120g arrowroot

1 tsp baking soda or powder

1 tsp ground cinnamon

½ cup / 50g chopped walnuts.

Method:

1. Combine water, raisins and dates in a 3 quart / 3.5 ltr saucepan. Boil for 10 minutes, then set aside to cool. Stir in the oil and lemon juice.

2. Into a medium bowl, sift the flour, arrowroot, baking soda and cinnamon. Stir the flour mixture into the saucepan, mix well, stir in the walnuts. Spread batter into an oiled 8" or 9" square baking pan. Bake at 400°F/200°C for 20 minutes, or until the top is firm when touched.

Pie Crust and Pies

Who doesn't like a pie – daft question!. This section includes a couple of recipes just for pastry so you can make your own choice of pie – and some health stores sell pastry ready-made which is wheat/ *Gluten free* – usually in the freezer.

Rice and Almond Flour Pie Crust Recipe

Gluten free

For sweet pies

Preheat oven to 350ºF/180ºC

Ingredients:

Grind 1/3rd cup / 50g whole almonds to a fine powder in a blender.

¾ cup / 95g brown rice flour

¼ tsp ground cinnamon

Pinch of ground cloves

3 tbs water

2 tbs light oil

2 tbs maple syrup

Method:

1.   In a bowl, combine the ground almond flour, brown rice flour, cinnamon or nutmeg and cloves. Mix well with a fork.
2.   In a pan, add the water, oil and maple syrup and heat on low setting until ingredients combine.
3.   3 Drizzle the Maple Syrup liquid over the flour mixture in the bowl, and stir with a fork until well blended. Let stand until the dry ingredients absorb the liquid.
4.   Shape the crust by pressing mixture firmly into place into a 9" pie dish with your fingers, covering bottom and sides of plate evenly. Pat top edge of crust into straight edge
5.   Bake before or after adding filling. Bake empty crust for 5 minutes at 350ºF/180ºC

Makes one crust. Note: Gluten-free dough will not toughen when handled

Pie Crust 2

Gluten free if not using barley flour

This recipe makes a single crust for a large pie

Ingredients:

1¼ cups / 190g barley, quinoa, or amaranth flour – you could mix flours for this recipe

1 tbs arrowroot powder

¼ teaspoon salt

3 tbs light oil

Method:

1.   Mix flour, arrowroot and salt in small mixing bowl. Add oil. Mix together well. Add 1 tbs cold water at a time, mixing after each addition until dough sticks together.
2.   Place dough on a piece of plastic wrap and flatten with your hands into a circle. Cover with another piece of plastic wrap and roll out to desired shape. Take one plastic piece off, and fit crust into pie pan, with the other plastic piece still on top. Finally, remove the second plastic piece. An alternative way to shape the dough is to simple press it into the pie dish with your fingers.

3. Prick pie crust with a fork, and bake for 20 mins at 350°F/180°C for a baked crust ready to be filled. For fruit or other mixtures, pre-cook crust at 350°F/180°C for 5 mins. so crust will stay flaky. Fill crust and bake as required.

Buckwheat Flour Pastry

Gluten free

This pastry is quick and easy to use, but you need to handle the rolled out pastry carefully. This pastry can be used for sweet or savoury fillings

For one 9 inch pie

Ingredients:

1 & ½ cups / 190g light buckwheat flour

¼ tsp salt

4 tbs light oil

Water – added gradually

Method:

Mix flour and salt in a mixing bowl. Add oil and mix, using fingers to mix oil with flour. Add water, 1 tablespoon at a time, until dough sticks together. Roll out half the dough at a time on a well-floured board. Carefully transfer one crust to the bottom of a 9 inch pie tin.

Bake at 400°F/200°C for 20 minutes, and then reduce temperature to 350°F/180°C and cook for an additional 15 minutes until golden brown.

Basic Crumble Topping

Small amount of gluten

Ingredients:

1¼ cups / 300g oats

1 tbs olive oil or lighter oil if preferred

1 tbs sunflower seeds

Method:

Preheat oven to 375°F/190°C. Mix together all ingredients. Sprinkle on top of filling and bake for 25 - 30 minutes, depending on the filling.

Millet Crumble Topping

Gluten free

Ingredients:

4 oz / 110g millet (or millet flakes)

2 cups / 500ml water

2 oz / 50g desiccated coconut (or freshly ground nuts)

Method:

1. Put the millet and water into a saucepan over a moderate heat, and simmer without stirring.
2. When water has been absorbed, turn off heat and place a lid on saucepan, allowing mixture to steam. Leave to cool, then add the coconut or ground nuts. Use in place of crumble topping for any recipe.

Buckwheat Berry Pie

Gluten free

One 9 inch pie

Ingredients:

1 & ½ cups/ 190g light buckwheat flour

¼ tsp salt

4 tbs light oil

1 cup / 250ml concentrated un-sweetened fruit juice, any flavour

2 tbs quick cooking tapioca

¼ tsp cinnamon (optional)

3 to 4 cups / 750 – 1000ml raspberries, blackberries, or other berries

Water

Method:

Preheat oven to 400°F/200°C

For the crust:

Mix flour and salt in a mixing bowl. Add oil and mix, using fingers to mix oil with flour. Add water, 1 tablespoon at a time, until dough sticks together. Roll out half the dough at a time on a well-floured board. Carefully transfer one crust to the bottom of a 9 inch pie tin.

For the filling:

Mix fruit and tapioca in a small saucepan. Bring to the boil and cook gently for 10 minutes, or until thick and clear and add the cinnamon.

Heap berries in a pie dish. Add fruit juice and tapioca mix. Carefully transfer the second crust to the top of the pie, cut a few holes for steam to escape, and flute the edge. Brush crust with a little milk and sprinkle with a little cinnamon.

Bake at 400°F/200°C for 20 minutes, then reduce temperature to 350°F/180°C and cook for an additional 15 minutes until golden brown.

Pizza Crust

Gluten free - yeast free

Ingredients:

½ cup/ 65g Garbanzo flour (chick-pea flour)

½ cup / 65g tapioca flour

1 tsp maple syrup

1 tsp Xanthan gum

½ tsp sea salt

¼ tbs agar-agar granules

½ tsp baking powder

½ tsp baking soda

½ onion powder

½ tsp crushed rosemary

½ tsp Italian herb blend

2 tsp egg replacement

½ cup/ 140ml milk (rice or nut milk)

1 tbs olive oil

Method:

Preheat oven to 400°F/200°C

Use a 12" non-stick pizza pan for a thin, crispy crust

Use a 10" cast iron skillet for a deep-dish crust

Prepare dish by spraying lightly with oil

1. In a small mixing bowl, combine all ingredients. Mix with electric mixer for 2 mins. Batter will be soft and sticky.
2. Spread batter in prepared pan, using a wet spatula to smooth the dough and push to, but not touching, the outer edges of pan. Make a little ridge around the edge to contain the pizza sauce and toppings.
3. Bake for 15 mins. Remove from oven, top with toppings and bake for another 10 mins. or until browned.

Makes 4 servings

Nut Base Pizza

Gluten free

Ingredients:

2 cups / 500ml nuts (macadamias, walnuts, hazelnuts, etc.)

3 tomatoes, sliced

2 cloves garlic, minced

1 sweet pepper, diced

1 courgette, sliced

1 cup / 75g mushrooms, sliced

1 onion, diced

1 cup / 100g pine nuts

1 teaspoon oregano

(plus any additional favourite herbs to your taste)

Olive oil

Method:

1. Preheat oven to 22°F/110°C.
2. Grind nuts into crumbs/mush using a blender or a food processor
3. Steam vegetables for 2-3 minutes (except for tomatoes).
4. Add ground nuts to a dish to form a base, then add vegetables on top. Drizzle some olive oil over top of pizza, and sprinkle oregano evenly on top.
5. Place pizza into oven and cook for 10 - 12 minutes. Garnish with pine nuts.

Serves 2 to 4 - Try experimenting with other vegetables, like sliced aubergine, sweet-corn.

Sauces, Dressings & Spreads for Sandwiches

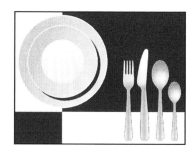

Sauces

These sauces can really expand your recipe list. Use them poured over freshly cooked vegetables. Mix your vegetables with pulses, beans, rice, wheat-free pastas, to make complete sustaining and nourishing meals. Many of the ingredients you will have in your cupboard already, so you only need to buy the few fresh ingredients to make a meal.

Basic Tomato Sauce/Juice

Since many classic recipes call for tomato juice or tomato sauce, it's good to know that you can make your own rather than rely on the canned varieties that contain additives. To make tomato juice, simply puree tomatoes in a blender, add lemon juice and salt. Strain the mixture for juice, and retain the pulp and a little juice to use in recipes calling for tomato sauce.

Good All Round Tomato Sauce

Makes about 2 pints

Ingredients:

4 tbs olive oil

2 onions

1 tsp dried oregano

1 tsp dried basil

1 tsp fennel seeds (optional)
4 garlic cloves, sliced

1 tsp ground black pepper

½ cup / 140ml tomato puree

1 carrot grated

1 small red or green pepper, finely chopped

2 cups / 500ml chopped tomatoes

1 tbs tamari

1/3rd cup / 160ml water

Method:

1. Soften together the onions and herbs in a heavy based saucepan with the oil.
2. Stir the tomato puree into the softened onion and heat for 3- 4 minutes, then add the rest of the ingredients. Stir well, lower the heat and simmer for 25 - 30 minutes.

Great on any kind of pasta or vegetables. Left to reduce and thicken, it makes a good pizza topping.

Rich Walnut Sauce

Ingredients:

2 garlic cloves

1 tbs tamari

½ cup / 140ml fresh basil leaves

1 generous cup/ 100g of walnuts

3 tbs cider vinegar

juice of 1 lemon

½ cup / 140ml chopped parsley

4-5 mint leaves

½ tsp ground black pepper

½ cup / 140ml olive oil

Method:

Whizz all ingredients until smooth in a blender.

This makes a good dip. If you like a bit of a 'kick', you could add fresh green chilli pepper to the sauce.

Bright Red Pepper (bell pepper) Sauce

Makes about 1 pint / 570ml

Ingredients:

2 garlic cloves

1 medium onion, shopped

3 red peppers, chopped

3 tbs olive oil

2 tsp tomato puree (paste)

Sea salt to taste

Pinch paprika

1 cup / 250ml water

Method:

1. Soften the vegetables in a little oil on a low heat. Add the remaining ingredients, stirring after each addition, adding the water last.

2. Reduce the heat, cover, and cook gently until the peppers are very soft, about 30 minutes. Let cool and whizz until smooth in a blender.

This sauce is delicious. It is wonderful with grains or pasta.

Mustard Sauce for Grilled Vegetables

Make sufficient to coat vegetables for 2 as a main course

Ingredients:

2 tbs yellow mustard seeds, soaked overnight in cider vinegar

2 tbs liquid sweetener

2 tbs tamari

1 tbs olive oil

Ground black pepper to taste

Method:

Whizz together in a blender

Spoon or spread this sauce on vegetables and grill for a tasty dish. Try it on: halved tomatoes, thin slices aubergine, thin slivers courgette, parsnip (par-boiled).

Coconut Cream Sauce

This sauce works really well poured over steamed vegetables like cabbage, broccoli, cauliflower, spinach, fish - in fact over just about anything.

Ingredients:

3 tbs sesame oil

1 small onion, finely chopped

2 garlic cloves, chopped

10 fl oz / 300ml coconut milk

¼ tsp Cajun seasoning (see below)

½ tsp ground turmeric

Sea salt

Freshly ground red pepper corns

2 tbs fresh coriander, finely chopped.

Method:

1. Put the oil into a pan and fry the onions and garlic until very light brown.

2. Add the coconut, all seasonings except coriander. Cook for 2 to 3 minutes, then remove from the heat.

3. Add fresh coriander and pour directly over vegetables, fish, whatever dish you are using sauce with.

Consider this sauce poured over freshly cooked pasta and steamed vegetable mixed together, for a complete meal.

Homemade Cajun seasoning

This seasoning is best made with fresh herbs. It will keep in the refrigerator for up to two weeks. If you want a dry mixture that will keep longer, use dried garlic and onion flakes.

Ingredients:

1 tsp paprika

½ tsp ground cumin

½ tsp fresh ground pepper

½ tsp mustard powder

½ tsp cayenne pepper

2 tsp fresh thyme or ½ tsp dried thyme

1 tsp sea salt

2 tsp fresh oregano or 1 tsp dried oregano

2-3 garlic cloves, well mashed

1 chilli, finely chopped

3 tbs onion, finely chopped

Method:

Combine all the ingredients by hand. Store in a jar with a tightly closing lid.

Curry and Herb Marinade

Ingredients:

3 cups / 750ml orange or yellow -

 pepper deseeded, and diced

¾ cup / 210ml white grape juice

1/3rd cup / 80ml shallots, finely chopped

1/3rd cup / 80ml lemon juice

1/3rd cup / 80ml olive oil

3 tbs tamari

4 tsp curry powder

¼ tsp salt

1/8th tsp pepper

1/3rd cup / 80ml freshly chopped basil

1/3rd cup 80ml freshly chopped parsley

Method:

In a blender, place all of the ingredients, except the chopped basil and parsley, and blend for 1-2 minutes or until thoroughly combined. Add the herbs and blend an additional 10 seconds. Transfer marinade to a bowl. Use as a marinade for vegetables or try as a dressing for salad.

Citrus and Herb Marinade

Ingredients:

2/3rds / 170ml cup lemon juice

½ cup / 150ml orange juice

1/3rd cup/ 80ml olive oil

¼ cup/ 70ml tamari

2 tbs freshly chopped parsley

1 tbs freshly chopped rosemary

2 tsp garlic, minced

1 tsp grated lemon zest

½ tsp salt

1/8th tsp freshly ground black pepper

Method:

In a small bowl, place all of the ingredients, and whisk well to combine. Use as a marinade for vegetables, or to add flavour to grains or pasta. Stores in an airtight container in the refrigerator for 5-7 days.

Dressings

Note: Some of these dressing contain different types of vinegar which needs to be kept to a minimum if you have a Candida issue. Vinegar can help to feed the candida overgrowth, but there are plenty of other dressings that are free of vinegar.

Lemon Vinaigrette

This versatile dressing enlivens almost any type of salad greens, beans or veggies. You can also use it as a simple sauce for cooked vegetables and meats, fish or poultry dishes – remember, you can have fish and poultry as long as it is organic and hopefully free from pollutants - The vinaigrette may be refrigerated for up to three days.

Ingredients:

3 tbs fresh lemon juice

1 large clove garlic

¾ tsp salt

½ tsp Dijon mustard

¼ cup / 80ml olive oil

Method:

Process lemon juice, garlic, salt and mustard in a blender on low speed. Gradually drizzle oil through feed tube, increasing speed to high until blended and smooth.

Parsley Vinaigrette

Makes about 1 pint / 570ml

Ingredients:

½ cup / 140ml olive oil

4 tbs cider vinegar

2 tbs tamari

1 tsp light tahini

Zest of 1 lemon

1 cup fresh parsley

Method:

Mix for a couple of minutes in a blender.

Vary this by using other herbs: try basil, mint or tarragon.

Lemon and Cumin Dressing

Makes about ½ pint / 280ml

Ingredients:

Juice and zest (finely grated rind) of 2 lemons

1 large, ripe tomato

2 garlic cloves

2 tsp cumin seeds, lightly toasted in a dry pan

1 tsp tamari

Pinch of paprika

2 tbs olive oil

1 tsp maple syrup or other liquid sweetener

1 tsp ground black pepper

Method:

Mix all ingredients together in a blender for a few minutes and it is ready to use.

Lovely for a grain salad. Also try it poured over cooked rice or rosti type dishes.

Fresh Tomato and Basil Dressing

Makes about ½ pint / 280ml

Ingredients:

2 large, fresh ripe tomatoes

2 tbs olive oil

1 tbs cider vinegar

Generous handful of fresh basil leaves.

Method:

Mix all ingredients in a blender until smooth.

Wonderful on cooked or raw vegetables/salad. Add a chopped red pepper (bell) for extra zing.

Orange and Sesame Dressing

Makes about ½ pint / 280ml

Ingredients:

Zest of 1 large orange, the segments chopped

1tbs cider vinegar

1 tbs tamari

1 tsp toasted sesame oil

1 tsp sesame seeds

2 tbs olive oil

Method:

Mix together in a blender.

Delicious on a mixture of finely shredded red and green cabbage, with sultanas and almonds.

Creamy Mint Dressing

Makes about 1 pint / 570ml

Ingredients:

4 tbs light tahini

2 tsp yellow mustard seeds, soaked overnight in cider vinegar

¼ pint / 140ml oil of choice

1 pint / 570ml cider vinegar

1 cup / 25g fresh mint leaves

1 tsp ground black pepper

1 tsp tamari

Method:

Mix all ingredients in a blender until smooth. Add a little water if it seems too thick to mix well.

Use this mix with loads of chopped cucumber and onion to make a dairy free raita to go with Indi-an-style dishes. Great on any salad dish or even spooned on baked potatoes with roasted roots veg

Zesty Dressing for salads

Mix together equal parts lemon juice, orange juice and lime juice.

Add fresh minced garlic, fresh dill and your favourite salad herbs

Pinch of sea salt

(can blend in avocado or olive oil if desired)

Chill to blend flavours

Serve over tossed salad

Jazzy Tahini Dressing

Ingredients:

¾ cup / 210ml sesame seeds soaked (3 hours) - blend seeds along with soak water until fairly smooth

Mix together with:

Juice of 1 lemon

Garlic to your taste

tbs or so ginger powder

½ cup / 140ml olive oil

Maple syrup to taste

About ¼ cup / 70ml apple juice

Tomato Vinaigrette

Ingredients:

2/3rds cup / 160 ml (approx) tomato juice (bottled from store – without added ingredients)

3 tsp balsamic vinegar

1 tbs wine vinegar

2 garlic cloves, crushed

1 tsp onion salt

10 leaves of fresh basil or tarragon

1 tbs tamari

Method:

Freshly ground black pepper

Blend all the ingredients together in a food processor or blender, then season to taste.

Olive Oil, Basil and Lemon Dressing

Ingredients:

2 tbs fresh lemon juice

5 tbs olive oil

Handful fresh basil leaves

1 tsp sea salt

Zest of ½ lemon, shredded fine

Freshly ground black pepper

Method:

Place all the ingredients except the lemon zest and pepper into a food processor or blender. Blend until smooth. Add the lemon zest and pepper and pour over salad.

Celery, shallot and tomato salad dressing/dip

Ingredients:

3 medium tomatoes, nice and ripe

4 oz / 110g fresh garden herbs of your choice

1 tbs sesame seeds

2 tbs lemon juice

Sea salt

Fresh ground black pepper

1 tbs shallots, finely chopped

¼ stick celery, finely chopped

Method:

Place all ingredients except shallots and celery in a food processor or blender and mix well. Remove mixture from processor to a dish, add the shallots and celery and stir.

Can be used as a dip or a dressing.

Tomato and Coriander Salsa

Makes about 2 cups / 500ml

Ingredients:

3 large, ripe tomatoes

1 onion or 6 spring onions

2 garlic cloves

1 cup / 30g fresh coriander leaves

½ tsp ground black pepper

Hot chilli pepper

Method:

Finely chop and mix all ingredients together or whizz for a couple of seconds in a blender. If you use a machine - start with the onions, then add the rest to process very briefly. If you over process you will end up with a soup rather than a salsa.

Dips and Spreads for Toast and Sandwiches

Nut Butter

Nut butters are very easily made in the food processor. Once made they can be thinned with a little oil and flavoured with herbs, spices and vegetables for savoury applications. They can also be mixed with fruit purees, chopped dates or bananas to make cake fillings, sweet spreads or fruit stuffings.

Suitable nuts are hazelnuts, walnuts and peanuts. Cashew nuts can also be used but they tend to remain much dryer without the addition of extra oil.

You need:

8 oz / 225g nuts

A little nut oil

Method:

Remove the skins from the nuts if necessary and blend in a food processor for a few minutes until the ground nuts start to exude their oils and stick together. Add a little more oil at this stage is necessary.

Fruit Butter

A less allergenic alternative to jams and jellies, using whatever fruit you wish.

Ingredients:

12 - 14 cups / 3 to 3 ½ ltrs chopped fruit

Water or un-sweetened juice or cider – to cover fruit

¼ cup / 70ml liquid sweetener

Method:

Place the fruit in pan, add enough water, juice or cider to cover, add the sweetener, bake at 275F/140c to 300 F /150c until fruit is mushy; do not allow to boil.

Puree the fruit in a processor or blender, taste and if necessary add more sweetener. Return to pot and bake again, stirring every 30 minutes, until very thick.

Ladle into sterile canning jars and seal tightly, place in a large pot and add enough water to cover the lids by an inch. Boil for 30 minutes. Cool, label and store at room temperature.

Sunflower Spread for Sandwiches or Toast

Makes about 1 pint / 570ml

Ingredients:

8 oz / 225g cooked green split peas, drained and cooled

1 generous tbs olive oil

1 cup / 250ml toasted sunflower seeds

3 tbs tamari (optional)

½ tsp ground black pepper

2 tbs lemon juice

½ tsp ground coriander

Method:

Grind the sunflower seeds in a food processor. Add the other ingredients and mix briefly to blend the mixture until you have a course pate.

You can vary this by adding a chopped and sautéed onion. Fresh root ginger is also good. Simply peel and chop pieces, sauté it with chopped onion and add to the mixture and mix with the other ingredients.

Red Bean Dip

Ingredients:

1 x 14 oz / 400g can red kidney beans, rinsed

½ tbs fresh lemon juice

1 - 2 cloves garlic depending on taste

1 tbs olive oil

1 tbs tomato puree

Method:

Put all ingredients together in a food processor or blender and mix. Serve as a dip or spread on hot toast for a snack. You could pile some chopped salad on top to make a lunch time sandwich. Will keep in the refrigerator for a few days, but keep it in a sealed container.

Avocado and Tomato Dip

Ingredients:

2 ripe avocados

1 large tomato, peeled

4 tbs fresh lemon juice

1 tbs chopped chives or spring onions

1 clove garlic, chopped

Method:

Peel and mash the avocado and tomato and thoroughly mix with the other ingredients.

Savoury Spread for Sandwiches or Toast

Makes about 1 pint

Ingredients:

1 cup / 250ml light tahini

1 cup / 250ml water

½ cup / 140ml tamari

1 tbs cider vinegar or lemon juice

Method:

Blend until thick and smooth. Keeps well in refrigerator.

No Bean Hummus

Ingredients:

2 medium courgettes

¼ cup / 70ml olive oil

4- 6 garlic cloves depending on taste

½ sea salt

½ cup / 40ml lemon or lime juice

¾ cup / 210ml sesame seeds

¾ cup / 210ml tahini

¼ tsp cayenne

1 tsp paprika

1 tsp ground cumin

Method:

Process courgettes, olive oil and garlic first in food processor or blender. Add remaining ingredients and process until smooth. Keeps well in refrigerator

Hummus (The chick-pea version)

Ingredients:

1 cup / 250ml chickpeas, soaked overnight and boiled for 1 hour OR

1 can sugar-free chickpeas, rinsed and drained

2 lemon, squeezed

1 tbs olive oil

1 - 2 garlic cloves, crushed (more if desired)

¾ cup / 100g ground sesame seeds

Method:

Puree chickpeas in a blender with the lemon juice and oil. Add garlic and ground sesame seeds, and mix to a thick paste adding water if necessary. Keep refrigerated.

Nut Pate

A blend of nutrition and taste

Ingredients:

1 cup / 150g almonds, soaked 12-48 hours and blanched

1 cup / 250ml sunflower seeds, soaked 6-8 hours and rinsed

¼ cup / 70ml sesame seeds, soaked 8 hours and rinsed

1 red bell pepper, finely chopped

3 stalks celery, finely chopped

1 small leek, finely chopped

1-2 tsp. powdered kelp

2 tbs lemon juice

Method:

Using a juicer or food processor process almonds, sunflower seeds, sesame seeds. Add red bell pepper, celery, leek, lemon juice, kelp, and mix well.

Keep refrigerated

Almond Pate

Ingredients:

Approx. 40 un-blanched whole almonds

½ stick celery

2 spring onions

1 small carrot

large squeeze lemon juice

2-3 tsp nori flakes (optional, or use other seaweed)

Method:

1. Soak the almonds at least overnight, or for up to 36 hours, changing the water every 12 hours.

2. Drain the almonds, and peel them if you can be bothered (I think it enhances the flavour).

3. Chop the celery and spring onions, peel and chop the carrot. Put these and the almonds into a blender, or food processor and process until smooth.

4. Add lemon juice to taste, and mix in the seaweed flakes. You could add salt if you want, but I don't think it needs it.

Lentil Pate

Ingredients:

1 medium onion

1 clove garlic

2 tbs olive oil

2/3rds / 150g cup lentils

2½ cups / 650ml vegetable stock

½ tsp ground turmeric

½ tsp ground coriander

½ tsp ground cumin

Method:

Chop the onion and garlic and soften in oil in a deep pan on a low heat. Rinse lentils and add to pan. Pour in stock and add spices. Bring to boil and then turn down heat, gently simmer until lentils are soft and the mixture is thick.

Remove from heat, leave to cool and then beat with a wooden spoon to make a pate, or alternatively use an electric mixer. Put into a glass dish ready to use.

Spicy Bean Pate

Ingredients:

1½ cups / 340ml pinto or aduki beans, soaked overnight

4 garlic cloves, peeled

1 large onion, finely chopped

2 garlic cloves, crushed

1 red pepper (bell), finely chopped

2 tbs olive oil

1 tsp ground cumin

1 tsp paprika

2 tsp tamari

Method:

1. Cook the beans with the 4 cloves of peeled garlic in water until the beans are very soft. When cooked, drain, mash with a fork or whizz in the blender.

2. Sauté the vegetables in the oil over a gentle heat until soft. Stir in the spices and garlic. Fry another few minutes. Add the tamari.

3. Stir the vegetable mix into the beans and press into 6 ramekins pots or a bowl. Cool.

Serve with hot bread (wheat-free of course) as a first course or chill and use as a sandwich filling.

Guacamole

This is the recipe for the Mexican avocado dish that works well as a dip for parties, and can also be used as the basis of a salad for your main meal.

Ingredients:

2 ripe avocados

2 tomatoes, peeled and finely chopped

6 spring onions, finely chopped

1 - 2 chillies, seeded and finely chopped

2 tbs fresh lime or lemon juice

1 tbs chopped fresh coriander

Sea salt to taste

Freshly ground black pepper

Method:

Put the avocado in a large bowl and mash them roughly with a fork.

1.   Add the remaining ingredients. Mix well and season according to taste and it is ready to serve.

Tips and Techniques

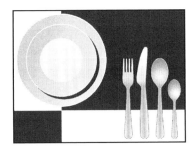

We will just finish off with a few helpful tips and techniques to assist you with your new diet .....

Almond Sprouts

When sprouting almonds, soak overnight, and sprout for 1 or 2 days. You will not be able to see the actual sprout unless you remove the skin, and then you will see it very clearly. Store them in the refrigerator in filtered water and change the water every two days to prevent fermentation. Keeps for up to a week.

Blanched Almonds
To remove the skins after sprouting

To blanche almonds (without cooking them), first prepare a large bowl of cold water into which you have added two trays of ice cubes. Then heat up some separate water to a boil, turn off the flame, and put in the sprouted almonds for 7 seconds. Time the 7 seconds, while stirring, and stay with the pot. If you move away to do something else, you might not come back to your almonds in the allotted time, and then you will have cooked them.

Drain the almonds quickly through a colander and plunge the colander into the ice water. This stops the process of cooking immediately. The almond skins will then pop off easily when you push them between your thumb and forefinger.

WHY IS IT NECESSARY TO REMOVE ALMOND SKINS? Almond skins have a high concentration of tannic acid. Research has indicated that tannic acid may interfere with the body's uptake of iron. When you eat a lot of almonds, it might be a good idea to remove the skins. (If you are just having a handful, then you don't need to skin them.)

Sprouting Seeds

Sprouted seeds and grains are simply packed with nutrients, vitamins and minerals. The vitamin content of seeds increases dramatically when they geminate. The vitamin B2 in an oat grain rises by 1300 per cent almost as soon as the seed sprouts, and by the time tiny leaves are formed, it has risen by 2000 per cent. Some sprouted seeds and grains are believed to have anti-cancer properties. Another attractive thing about sprouts is their price.

The basic seeds and grains are cheap and readily available in supermarkets and health stores - chickpeas, brown lentils, mung beans, alfalfa etc. You can sprout them yourself, and all you have to add is fresh water. You then have easily accessible, organically grown fresh sprouts that are packed full of nutrients.

Sprouting is easily done, and once germinated can be kept in the refrigerator in polythene bags for up to a week. Most people grow sprouts in glass jars covered with nylon mesh held in place with an elastic band around the neck. You can also buy special sprouting containers from health-shops.

Here's how to sprout seeds

Place two handfuls of seeds or beans in the bottom of a jar or bowl and cover with plenty of water - use at least one part seed to three parts water. Leave to soak overnight.

Pour the seeds into a sieve and rinse well with water. Be sure to remove any dead or broken seeds. If you are using glass jars then return the soaked seeds to the jar after rinsing well and cover with cheesecloth secured with a rubber band, drain well and keep in a warm dark place. They can even be covered with a bag or a cloth to create darkness.

Rinse thoroughly twice a day and be sure to drain them well or you will find they may become mouldy.

While they are sprouting, the hulls of some seeds come off - usually while you are rinsing them. Discard the hulls as they tend to rot easily. You can do this by placing the sprouts in a big bowl of water and shaking it gently to separate the hulls from the sprouts themselves. Usually the hulls sink to the bottom.

After about three days, place the seeds in sunlight for several hours to develop the chlorophyll in them. Rinse in a sieve, drain well and put in a polythene bag in the refrigerator to use in salads, stir-fries etc.

There are many different seeds you can sprout, each with its own particular flavour and texture. Some sprouts, such as radish or mustard are zesty and add fire to a dish. They mix well with milder sprouts such as alfalfa or mung.

Utensils

The implements you use when cooking can affect health. Rinse detergents thoroughly from kitchenware, since experiments have linked them with eczema and damage to the intestinal lining. Earthenware pots are sometimes glazed with lead or cadmium, which can be dangerous. White porcelain or glass containers are more suitable. Copper, brass or aluminium pans should be avoided. Aluminium, especially, may be associated with digestive-system complaints ranging from mouth ulcers to piles. Aluminium in the system has also been associated with Alzheimer's disease. Non-stick teflon coatings may lead to gut ulcers when they start to peel off.

Stainless steel pans are suitable, especially if they have the copper insert, sandwiched in the bottom, as this allows quick and even distribution of heat. Iron utensils are recommended since they distribute heat evenly for thorough cooking, and they may also be a source of iron in the diet.

Beans and Pulses - dried or tinned!

In the recipes in this book, I have alternated between using dried beans and tinned beans. There are many beans that now come ready cooked and sold in tins, including chick peas, kidney beans, black eye beans, to name a few.

In an ideal world you should really cook all your own beans but this may not be practical or economical. If for instance you only need ½ a cup of beans for a salad recipe, then it is ridiculous to cook your own beans. If you are good at planning meals in advance then you could cook a 'job lot' of beans and utilise them in 2 or 3 recipes – you could freeze beans that you have cooked but just make sure you get them as dry as possible before putting them in the freezer otherwise they will crack and go a bit mushy when thawing.

My advice is to use your common sense. You do not want to be 'busting a gut' to feed yourself. Do use tinned beans when the need arises but give them a rinse to get rid of any sugar that may have been added.

Using Yoghurt in your Cooking

As with the bean issue above, I have alternated between using nut yoghurt and natural yoghurt in some recipes. The choice is really up to you and if you want to totally eliminate yoghurt from your diet then use a nut yoghurt. As I mentioned in the introduction, 'live' natural yoghurt is actually beneficial for your intestinal flora, so feel free to use it.

Note. When using yoghurt in cooking, blend ½ teaspoon of cornflower to yoghurt before adding to pan and heat gently, stirring constantly. The cornflower helps stabilise the yoghurt to prevent it separating during heating.

Ideas for snacks

We all feel like snacking at times, but most of us snack on chocolate bars, biscuits and other unhealthy nibbles. Here are few suggestions to give you something healthy to snack on - you could have nuts, dried fruit, fruit and nut mix, rice cakes and dips, crispbreads and dips, fresh fruit, flapjack bars or similar health bars. You may find other nice snack foods in your local health shop, both sweet and savoury.

Shopping List

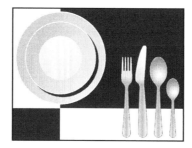

Your stock cupboard supplies for the recipes in this book – these are the basics and you will no doubt add to these as you go along.

Dry Foods

*   Sweeteners - stevia, maple syrup, rice syrup and others you wish to try
*   Selection of herb teas – camomile, fennel and peppermint are all great for the digestive system
*   Green Tea – caffeine free
*   Gluten free muesli and breakfast cereals
*   Cacao powder - see the endo-friendly chocolate recipe for ideas
*   Rice noodles
*   Wheat/Gluten free pasta selection
*   Rice - brown and basmati
*   Various Gluten free flours - depending on what you want to cook from the recipes
*   All-round Gluten free flour which gives you quick flexibility
*   Gluten free rice cakes or crackers
*   Corn flour - to thicken sauces
*   Almond flour - which is basically ground almonds and used a lot here
*   Baking powder
*   Almonds and other nuts of your choice
*   Dried organic fruit selection
*   Dried pulses and lentils of your choice - there are loads of them
*   Tins of: coconut milk, tinned plumb tomatoes - they sell organic varieties in health stores - a good staple to add to casseroles, tinned chickpeas/garbanzo's, kidney beans - again available in health stores with no added salt or sugar
*   Seeds – sesame, sunflower, pumpkin – great for snacking on
*   Lots of different herbs and spices

Liquid Foods

*   Olive oil - a good quality, extra virgin, cold pressed
*   Nut oils, sesame oil, rapeseed oil for cooking
*   Nut butter (try the ones available in the health store)
*   Lemon juice - a good standby to have
*   Coconut milk - available in tins and a thinner version in cartons
*   Rice wine vinegar - good for dressings
*   Apple cider vinegar - has plenty of health benefits
*   Tamari - the alternative to soy sauce
*   Tahini - similar to peanut butter but made from ground sesame seeds and is used in lots of recipes here
*   Tubes of tomato puree

Health food stores

Have a good look round. These stores are now selling items like - gluten/wheat free breakfast cereals, Almond milks, Rice milk, Coconut milk, breakfast/mid-morning snacks. Some stores also sell ready meals, alternative spreads for toast like mushroom paste. Just ensure to check ingredients for soy proteins, wheat powder/flour and gluten.

Other ingredients

The other items you need will be purchased as and when you need them, like fresh produce, fruit, and vegetables. I am not against using frozen vegetables as these maintain a reasonable level of nutritional value, but aim to purchase from the freezer in your health store as these should be organic and not covered in sprays and pesticides etc.

Other items you might need

Get a supply of those little freezer trays/containers with lids for freezing separate portions to use later when you have done any bulk cooking. A pestle and mortar is great to have for grinding up spices and nuts - makes you feel like a proper chef using one of these!

Food processor - takes the hard work out of the preparation for some recipes

If you can afford it a juice extractor is great - then you can have freshly made juice that does not waste any of the fruit, and obtains as many nutrients and enzymes as possible.

Last word

Taking on a diet like this is going to take a while for you to adjust. You will need to re-stock your cupboards; learn slightly different cooking skills, especially when preparing the 'raw' foods. You will have to break some very old and ingrained habits.

Do not try and do it all at once. Do a little at a time. Maybe set yourself tangible, weekly targets. For example:

- Week one - change your hot drinks intake and change over to healthy options
- Week two - change your lunch-time habit of having a wheat based sandwich every week day - change over to a healthy alternative, like buying an alternative to wheat bread from your health store and adding some healthy dips and salad
- Week three - be brave and chuck out all those nasty ingredients from your cup-boards and restock with safer alternatives
- Week four - start to write up meal plans, building in time-tables for your periods so you can plan what to cook in advance to get you through rough times
- Week five - gradually build up your new diet regime to include all meals based on the Endo diet
- Week six - continue building this new regime. Do not worry about lapses, you are only human. In a few weeks' time you will be able to detect what really upsets your system when you have a relapse. I think wheat and coffee will knock your system side-ways - it does for a lot of women
- At around week ten - give yourself a huge treat - go for a lovely therapeutic mas-sage if you can afford it. If you can't afford a trained masseur, then maybe a friend who has a natural touch could give you one. Whatever you do, don't throw in the towel. The benefits will not come over night, but they will come. Believe me, many women have had huge benefits from changing their diet and have reduced their endometriosis symptoms immensely.

Yours with healing thoughts

Carolyn Levett

www.endo-resolved.com

Index

Additional Reading

This book – by its very title - is a recipe book but as you have read, there is plenty of background information in the introduction to back-up the advice. Even so, there is plenty more advice that can be given about diet, nutrition, digestion, digestive health, detox etc. – so I felt it simpler to add that information as links direct to the website at www.endo-resolved.com You can then read these pages in your own time.

The Endometriosis Nutrition & Diet Glossary – This mini e-book has been put together to give you more knowledge about the role of diet and nutrition in relation to endometriosis. It is compiled as a detailed A to Z glossary - to help you with your research, and learn more about nutrition and how it assists with your health. There is also advice on all the various supplements, vitamins and minerals. You can download the e-book direct from here: http://www.endo-resolved.com/support-files/diet_nutrition_endometriosis.pdf

Constipation - Here is my personal view on constipation, with my personal experience, and some advice on how to deal with it. You can find an article about it here: http://www.endo-resolved.com/endometriosis_constipation.html

Toxic toiletries - To find out more about toxic toiletries and how to avoid them – you will find lots more advice here: http://www.endo-resolved.com/toiletries.html

Whole-grains - and gluten free whole-grains – a brief article explaining what whole grains are and how to incorporate more of them in your diet. You can find the article here: http://www.endo-resolved.com/whole_grains.html

Calcium intake – some women are concerned they may not have sufficient calcium in their diet if they remove dairy foods. There are plenty of other sources of calcium and you can find that advice here: http://www.endo-resolved.com/endometriosis_diet_calcium.html

As long as the website is 'Alive and kicking' then these links will be available, and your purchase of this book will help to keep the website going into the future. Thanks

References:

'Endometriosis – A key to Healing and Fertility through Nutrition' by Dian Shepperson Mills & Michael Vernon - 2002

'What Your Doctor May Not Tell You about Premenopause' by Dr. John Lee

'Quantum Healing' by Deepak Chopra – 1990

'The Coconut Oil Miracle' by Bruce Fife – 2004

'The Body Ecology Diet: Recovering Your Health and Rebuilding Your Immunity' by Donna Gates